# The Fertile Secret

## 10 Steps to Living Your Most Fertile Life

By Dr. Robert Kiltz

With
Kathryn Simmons Flynn

"The doctor of the future will give no medicines, but will interest his patients in the care of the human frame, in diet, and in the causes of disease."

— Thomas Edison

Published by Goat House Books in the United States of America.



ISBN: 0983845824
ISBN-13: 978-0-9838458-2-9

Goat House Books Printing, July 2013

Illustrations by Coburn Design

Edited by Jessie Briel

"The Fertile Secret is a medically accurate guide to becoming healthy and fertile on all levels. I applaud Dr. Kiltz on this wonderful approach to healing."

— Christiane Northrup, M.D, *Ob/gyn physician and author of the New York Times bestsellers: Women's Bodies, Women's Wisdom and The Wisdom of Menopause*

"I'm so happy to finally have a holistic fertility book to refer my readers to that combines the best of both eastern and western medicine. With its stress on the mind/body connection, it helps couples to achieve balance in their lives while pursuing their dream of conceiving."

— Toni Weschler, *MPH and author of both Taking Charge of Your Fertility and Cycle Savvy*

"If you are holding The Fertile Secret in your hands right now, perhaps your journey to create your family has taken you down a road that you didn't necessarily expect. The Fertile Secret is a compilation of information about the balancing of the mind, body and spirit. Be at peace now that you have this amazing content all in one place to read, re-read and help you answer the many questions you are likely to have on this journey."

— Kristen Magnacca, *Author of Girlfriend To Girlfriend: A Fertility Companion and Love & Infertility: Survival Strategies for Balancing Infertility, Marriage and Life*

## Praise for Dr. Rob Kiltz, his CNY Fertility and CNY Healing Arts Staff

"If it weren't for Dr. Rob looking outside the box and telling me not to give up, on what seemed to be the impossible, then my mornings would not consist of the beautiful smile that melts my heart when I walk into my daughter's room. I would not have those little "strong" arms grabbing me around my neck to hug me. I wouldn't hear the squeals of laughter from down the hall as she lets me know "Mommy, I am awake now." I thank God everyday for this precious gift to my life. I thank CNY Fertility for giving me the only chance I would have had to be a Mom. The staff made me feel like they knew me my entire life from day one, and it was hard to say goodbye. I will always be grateful to you all! I have learned through this that if there is even the slightest chance, giving up should not be an option! You just have to believe it can happen, visualize it, dream it, and without doubt, you will achieve it."

— Paula

"We have been trying to figure out the words to express our gratitude we have for Dr. Kiltz and his whole staff up at CNY Fertility. I have never met such friendly caring staff. They made me feel very positive about everything and were truly some of the nicest people I have come across. I was referred to Dr.Kiltz from my OB/GYN after laparoscopic surgery determined I had stage 4 endometriosis. I started with injections of Lupron and Gonal F for IVF. The first round did not work out, my levels were too high so we had to wait a month and then try again. This time it worked. On October 30th, I had my beautiful 7 lb., 8 oz. baby girl. I could never fully express the thanks I have for everyone at CNY. But thank you, Dr. Rob and everyone, for all your help and support!"

— Colleen and Daniel

"I want to thank you for making my dreams come true. Throughout the whole process I kept very positive about getting pregnant, but when my husband and I met you, it made me feel like this was really going to happen for me. I knew I was finally going to be a mother. You made us feel so comfortable, and you assured us that we were going to have babies; not one, but two. I am happy to tell you that I am 22 weeks pregnant with a baby boy. I thank you for making my dreams come true."

— Brenda and Enrique

"It would be eight Christmases and eight IVF procedures, along with an emotional ride that nearly destroyed us. Throughout everything we found such encouragement and sincerity at a soulful level from Rob. He truly could feel our pain and worked painstakingly with us, as though we were his only patients, which by now, he had moved on his own and was working 22hrs a day to keep up with every new patient. Because, with Rob, every patient is treated like they are the only patient. Rob laughed and cried with us when the news was confirmed. Nine months later, the most precious GIFT was bestowed on Suzanne and me. Maxwell, our First Born, had arrived. There is nothing in this world I would take over that GIFT, made possible through the life energy gifted to Rob.

Four years later and an incredible 4 year old, the Universe GIFTED us, unassisted, our angelic Emily. We still believe Rob put in a word with the Universe on our behalf. Max and Emily are now 8 and 4, I have happily decided that someday Max will drive me around in his Corvette."

— Endless Joy

"Almost one year ago to the day I met you and my life changed forever. For two years my husband and I tried to have a baby and just when it was beginning to look hopeless we were referred to

CNY Fertility. On March 19 I gave birth to two beautiful healthy baby boys, Patrick Gregory 6lbs 5oz and Gabriel Bosco 5lbs 14 oz. Thanking you does not even seem enough for what you have given me but it is all I can give. I lived in Albany and when I was pregnant I met people that you helped there and now that we are back in Rochester I continue to meet people here that you help as well.
You are a wonderful person and I hope that you always have your unfailing energy and optimism. Thank you for giving me mine."

— Jillian

"We tried to get pregnant on our own for almost 2 years. After 2 unsuccessful IUI's and clomid rounds with my OB/GYN, we turned to Dr. Kiltz and the CNY Fertility Center in Dec 2005. Dr. Kiltz wasted no time in trying to find the problem. In Jan 2006 I had a laparoscopy and stage 2 endometriosis was removed. That next cycle we started injections and thus became pregnant with twins!"

— CNY Fertility Client

"After nearly 2 years of unsuccessful fertility treatments at another fertility center, my husband and I came to CNY Fertility and thanks to Dr. Rob we are now pregnant with our first child (a girl). We are due April 1st and are so happy!! Thank you so much Dr. Rob!!!"

— Elise

"On February 13th, you held our hands and asked us to think positive thoughts as you retrieved the little follicle that would become the greatest gift we've ever been given. I must admit, after many unsuccessful attempts, I was skeptical. Karen & I knew all too well the disappointment of attempts that "didn't take" and were hardly consoled as we watched those around us succeed, when we only failed.

Everything changed for us on that February day. We "drank the kool-aid" and stayed positive all weekend. After the subsequent embryo transfer, I confined her to bed and waited on her hand and foot, trying to keep her relaxed while we kept positive thoughts. Through the weeks of bed rest that followed, we experienced moments of total kindness. Friends and strangers alike prayed for us, offered us their energy, one woman even offered to carry a child for us! An incredible, if not unbelievably awkward, gesture. I read your emails aloud to Karen and we regularly drove to acupuncture. I TRULY BELIEVE that made the difference. Karen was so relaxed; I thought she'd been drugged. I'd never seen her so stress free.

When I realized the acupuncture had worked its charms, I knew this was our chance.

On October 23rd, Mason Robert arrived. Two and a half weeks early and years in the making. I cannot thank you or your staff enough. You have honestly changed our lives forever. Thank you, thank you, thank you!"

—Jeff & Karen

"One year ago, I was in complete disbelief that I was pregnant. It had already been a long and trying road before I had that positive beta. We had lost two pregnancies in the five years prior. After trying for several years, Dr. Kiltz started me with gonal-f after I did not respond to clomid or femera. Gonal-f and an IUI with prometrium, lovenox, and several other medications got us to a positive beta. I didn't believe that it would "stick". Throughout the process, my friends from real life and online kept positive thoughts for me. In January of 2009, we welcomed our son into our life. He is the light of our life, and we thank Dr. Kiltz and the staff at CNY Fertility Center in Syracuse, NY for helping to bring him to us."

— CNY Fertility Client

"After changing clinics, I met with Dr. Kiltz at

CNY Fertility. During my consultation I explained my journey (3 Fresh IVF cycles & 4 Frozen all failed) he asked if he could examine me (right then and there!!!). After my examination, he explained that my fallopian tubes may be full of hydrosalpinx and that could be the reason why the embryo's weren't sticking. He wanted to check and make sure: if his theory was correct, he would suggest removing my tubes and going through another fresh cycle with CNY Fertility. Removing my tubes was the best thing he could have ever done for me. Not only do I no longer suffer from painful menstruation periods, my very next fresh (4th IVF) cycle resulted in a live birth. Cooper Daniel was born July 20, 2007."

— CNY Fertility Client

"After more than 3 years of trying to have a baby we finally found Dr. Kiltz through our GP. After two failed IVF's we were ready to give up, the heartbreak was more than we could bear, but Dr. Rob was not ready to give up. He told us about an experimental treatment called IVIG. Since we decided we were only going to try one more time, why not try it? Well it worked, and we welcomed a beautiful little girl into our world just before Valentine's Day! We cannot express in words the joy we feel or the lifetime of love that we have been blessed with. Thank you Dr. Kiltz, your belief that dreams come true is infectious and the positive vibes that you project are truly addictive. We are still numb, yet every time we look at our baby we melt!"

— CNY Fertility Client

"We would like to thank CNY Fertility Center for the amazing work they do everyday. After being diagnosed with PCOS and three failed rounds of clomid, we went to CNY. In April of 2008 we were pregnant, and in December 2008 we had a beautiful baby girl. Dr. Kiltz and his staff are amazing! CNY Fertility and CNY Healing Arts are places of hope, love and support. We will always have a special place in our heart for CNY and we are thankful everyday for the blessing of our daughter! She is a miracle, and we are so thankful!!! Thank you everyone at CNY!!!!"

— Shannon

"Thank you for making our dream of having a baby come true. After 2 miscarriages (and being a little older) we started to wonder if our dream of having a baby would ever come true. We were referred to your office by our family practitioner and felt comfortable with you and your staff from the moment we walked in your office. You all treated us with such kindness and explained the procedures in detail. The IUI worked on the first try, and all of your careful monitoring of the first precious weeks paid off. We feel so blessed. Thank you! You and your team are the best!!!"

— CNY Fertility Client

"I will never forget that feeling I experienced once those babies were placed in my arms in the recovery room that beautiful morning. All the feelings of fear, stress, anxiety, sadness, hurt, and anger that built up over the 3 years prior while we struggled with the challenges we faced with infertility were washed away in a tidal wave of tears. At one time it was so difficult to imagine this moment, as it seemed it might never happen. And all of the sudden here it was, here they were: our beautiful babies.

Dr Kiltz created a miracle for us that day. He creates miracles for so many people. Thank you for a day I will never forget. Every time I read your daily intentions, I bring myself back to that day and remind myself of the reason I was put on this earth…to be a great mom. When becoming a mom seemed so impossible--too much of a challenge for me to handle--you and your wonderful staff were there to show me the way. All our Love!"

— Allyson, Frank, Nicolas & Francesca

"Thank you, Dr. Kiltz, and all the staff at CNY Fertility. After trying for over 2 years to get pregnant and dealing with endometriosis, surgery and treatments, we met with you and came up with a plan. Five months later, we were pregnant. On December 18th, 2007 we welcomed our little boy. We are blessed and grateful to you. We are looking forward to seeing you all again soon."

— Brandon, Mary & Hayden

"CNY Fertility Center certainly made all of our dreams come true! At our first consultation, we went in with pre-conceived ideas of how to proceed, but the nurses, Dr. Kiltz, and the financial "guru" discussed all of our options, and it turned out that IVF offered the best option for us to start with. From that first meeting, we never questioned the advice of the staff, and were happier with that advice than ANY outcome we would have gotten from our initial plan. We were lucky enough that our first attempt at IVF was a success, and are loving life with our wonderful daughter!

I can't say enough about the patient experience at CNY Fertility. From the décor to the friendly, knowledgeable staff and caring medical professionals, CNY went WAY beyond typical medical intervention. I was so happy to be able to explore acupuncture and other alternative methods during my IVF journey – methods that may have been ignored, questioned, or discouraged elsewhere. Even though we have since moved away from central NY, if/when we decide to expand our family, there is no question that I would travel to the ends of the earth to work with CNY Fertility Center again."

— CNY Fertility Client

*This book is dedicated to my mother, Maria,*
*and my father, Raymond, for their*
*love and guidance and the gifts that they have bestowed upon*
*me in my life.*
-R.K.

*To my father, Rob Simmons, thank you for teaching me the*
*art of patience and perseverance and for being an infinite*
*source of wisdom in my life.*
*-K.S.F.*

# Foreword

It is my privilege to introduce Dr. Robert Kiltz's book, *The Fertile Secret: 10 Steps to Living Your Most Fertile Life*. I have been blessed by having Dr. Robert Kiltz in my life in so many ways: from his generosity of spirit to his "lead by example" approach to his life and work. Dr. Rob doesn't ask of others what he is not willing to do himself.

The example that strikes me most is his intention of becoming more "fertile", if you will, by continuing to be loving, forgiving and open-hearted each and everyday through his practice at CNY Fertility & CNY Healing Arts Center, and now through *The Fertile Secret*.

*The Fertile Secret* is a compilation of information about the balancing of the mind, body, and spirit, to create your heart's desire. It offers different options as you move through the journey to create a family, wholeness, or to rebirth yourself. This book offers you different options to integrate into your journey. Integration is another theme in Dr. Rob's philosophy. He looks at the "whole" of the person and works with his clients to grow and achieve success through their life lessons.

*The Fertile Secret* offers Western Medical definitions to physical conditions and teaches how the blending of Eastern and Western approaches will ease your mind and body. Over two years ago, when I met Dr. Rob, we were driving on our way to an event at one of his facilities. In the course of our conversation, I asked him a simple question.

"Do you set your intention before you enter into an appointment with your clients?"

Now, you must already be getting the idea that Dr. Rob is not your typical reproductive endocrinologist.

He asked me in return, "What do you mean?"

"When you pick up a chart, before entering the room, do you set a 'mini-goal' of how you want the meeting to go for your client?" I clarified.

We discussed this concept of setting an "intention" with clients. Dr. Rob integrated this concept into his life, his work, and his teaching. Here, he lead me by example, teaching me how to take a moment from a busy day and connect with the divine part of you, opening up a fountain of love for all.

What I mean by this is best described with an experience I witnessed at CNY Fertility & Healing Arts Center.

It was a Saturday morning in the Latham, NY Center and I was organizing the waiting area in the clinic for my presentation to Dr. Rob's Clients. He invited me to share my experience with our "Fertility Challenges" along with the strategies throughout my book, *Love and Infertility: Balancing Infertility, Marriage and Life*, with his clients.

The beautiful lobby had plush chairs and pillows. The warm fire from the fireplace was crackling, and the lights were softly shining when I struck up a conversation with the only person in the room.

He was waiting for his wife after they had an IVF transfer. I could feel his anxiety level as I opened the large bag of chocolates for the seminar attendees and offered him one. As he munched the chocolates, the lobby door swung open. It was one of the CNY Healing Arts staff members from upstairs. She looked at the husband and said:

"You know what? Our massage therapist has a little break. Why don't you come up and see her and wait upstairs for your wife?"

Off they both went up the stairs. Within seconds the door to the clinic opened and his wife appeared. She was wearing a white fluffy robe with matching slippers, the nurse had her hand on the middle of her back, supporting her ever so gently when she walked. They stopped for a moment for the nurse to make her a cup of tea and she escorted her upstairs for an acupuncture appointment.

These small acts of support were not done with

fan-fare or proclamations. They were just intended and done to support the clients as they move forward through this journey. Here is the big part: supporting the WHOLE of these patients, both partners, the individual person, the mind, body and soul of the person, and their approach to this situation: from the "Western Medical" to the "Eastern Approach" for the benefit of the whole.

I sat in the waiting room alone and cried. The intention of creating an environment of love and support was integrated into all systems of Dr. Kiltz's clinic long before our conversation on intention. He just made it public by sending out his daily intentions through his words.

*The Fertile Secret* is another vehicle for Dr. Rob's intention and passion for healing to be shared. If you are holding *The Fertile Secret* in your hands right now, perhaps your journey to create your family has taken you down a road that you didn't necessarily expect.

Be at peace now that you have this amazing compilation of information in one place to read, re-read, and help you answer the many questions you are likely to have on this journey.

Blessings,

Kristen Magnacca

# Preface

As a reproductive endocrinologist, I work with many men and women who experience a deep desperation for a child. In times where couples feel challenged to conceive, I have witnessed many feelings of hopelessness and talk of failures. A diagnosis of infertility often brings with it fear (a deep contraction), as we are overwhelmed with a multitude of emotions from guilt to shock to shame. By learning to release the constriction in your own body, you allow yourself to open to the unlimited possibilities available to you in this present moment. With this simple shift, you can open yourself to living your most fertile life.

In order to find the place of receptivity and deep healing, each client's feelings and innermost needs must be addressed. I believe that the relationship between a doctor and a client is a partnership that we navigate together, both holding the intention of creating greater health. This is the place where Western medicine and complementary medicine can work together to align the mind and the body, with the ultimate goal of improving life quality, even beyond the fertility journey.

*The Fertile Secret* is within each of us. By finding the place of peace and balance amidst the demands of life and the stress of infertility, we can renew our life-giving potential. Within this book's pages, I will introduce you to an integrative approach to treating infertility through concepts, exercises, and tools intended to support you in living your most fertile life.

Step out and create your life. Tap into the spiritual energy of this amazing life. And most of all send out love, love, and more love, to everyone!

Dr. Rob

# Contents

# Step 1:
# Explore Emotional Infertility

"Fertility is a lifelong relationship with oneself- not a medical condition."
— Joan Borysenko, PhD

## The diagnosis of infertility

In life, we are often thrown curve balls we do not expect or necessarily desire. When we embark on the fertility journey, most of us assume it's just a matter of time, and the process of conception will be fairly easy. In truth, the chance of conceiving in any given month is not as high as one might believe. With all of the intricate aspects that must come into play, a couple has a twenty-five percent chance of conceiving each month. For some, the fertility journey becomes a winding road where they must overcome various physical and emotional challenges for conception to occur. In fact, 7.3 million couples in the United States, or roughly 10% of the population of reproductive age, face the diagnosis of infertility: the inability to conceive after one year of regular unprotected intercourse (6 months in women over the age of 35).[i] This diagnosis can leave a couple absolutely devastated.

Dr. Alice Domar, Director of the Mind/Body

Center for Women's Health at Boston IVF, has conducted pioneering research on the impacts of stress and fertility. Her studies have shown that women facing infertility experience depression equivalent to those diagnosed with terminal illnesses like cancer.[ii] Some women literally feel as though their bodies have turned against them, and many couples spiral into the deepest levels of despair in a vicious cycle of disappointment, sadness, grief and frustration. When our bodies do not "perform" as we believe they should, it becomes harder to reside in the place of receptivity. At this point, couples can become increasingly negative in their emotions, thoughts and feelings. I have observed many clients in this exact cycle. In order to heal the physical and emotional elements of fertility, we must address the relationship between the mind and the body. By shifting the mind's relationship to the diagnosis of infertility, I have seen many couples heal physical imbalances and overcome seemingly irreversible diagnoses.

Mind-body medicine is revealing the ability within each of us to re-examine our deepest held beliefs and reveal our unlimited potential to heal ourselves. This is an amazing compliment to Western medical treatments, as it gives clients tangible methods of reducing stress and anxiety, creating the opportunity for more peace and serenity. When we begin to see the opportunity behind every perceived disappointment, we open ourselves to limitless possibilities for healing.

"The mind/body approach to fertility is based on the premise that knowledge is power and that a change in perception based on new information is powerful enough to effect subtle changes in your endocrine, immune, and nervous systems. Regardless of what you've been told about your fertility, you need to know that your ability to conceive is profoundly influenced by the complex interaction among psychosocial, psychological, and emotional factors, and that you can consciously work with this to enhance your ability to have a baby." [iii]
— Dr. Christiane Northrup

## The physiology of stress in your body

There is no debate that increased levels of stress contribute to illness, from increased blood pressure to digestive disturbances and lowered immune function. More recently, researchers have shown a direct link between increased stress hormones with menstrual cycle disturbances, ovulatory dysfunction, uterine receptivity and tubal function.[iv] Physiologically, stress hormones, including cortisol, ACTH, nor epinephrine and epinephrine are released into the bloodstream by the sympathetic nervous system and hypothalamic-pituitary-adrenal axis, forcing the body into "survival mode".[v] In a state of "fight or flight", vital functions are prioritized over reproductive function. This is most obvious as seen in animals in the wild. When an animal is in danger, reproductive function literally shuts down in favor of vital functions like the heartbeat. When we become stressed by perceived threats, our bodies react in the same way, by releasing a steady flow of stress chemicals. In Gabor Mate's book, *When the Body Says No*, he states that, "the body's hormonal system is inextricably linked with the brain centers where emotions are experienced and interpreted. In turn, the hormonal apparatus and the emotional centers are interconnected with the immune system and the nervous system. These are not four separate systems, but one super-system that functions as a unit to protect the body super-system from external invasion and from disturbances to the internal physiological condition. It is impossible for any stressful stimulus, chronic or acute, to act on only one part of the super-system."[vi]

To restore health and reduce stress we must learn to reverse "fight or flight" instantly, and protect our nervous systems. In an age where we process more information in one day than our ancestors did in an entire lifetime, the challenge is to find time to go within. Choosing activities that bring us a sense of peace and calm reduces the harmful effects of stress hormones. These activities elicit the "relaxation response," a technique discovered by Harvard cardiologist Dr. Herbert Benson in the early 1970s.[vii] While the "stress response" is instinctive, the relaxation response can be achieved by practicing techniques such as yoga, meditation, breath work and visualizations.

Herbert Benson's Steps to Elicit the Relaxation Response[viii]

This relaxation technique is being reprinted with permission from Dr. Herbert Benson's book, *The Relaxation Response*, pages 162-163.

**1.** Sit quietly in a comfortable position.
**2.** Close your eyes.
**3.** Deeply relax all your muscles, beginning at your feet and progressing up to your face. Keep them relaxed.
**4.** Breathe through your nose. Become aware of your breathing. As you breathe out, say the word "one"* silently to yourself. For example, breathe in ... out, "one,"- in ... out, "one," etc. Breathe easily and naturally.
**5.** Continue for 10 to 20 minutes. You may open your eyes to check the time, but do not use an alarm. When you finish, sit quietly for several minutes, at first with your eyes closed and later with your eyes opened. Do not stand up for a few minutes.
**6.** Do not worry about whether you are successful in achieving a deep level of relaxation. Maintain a passive attitude and permit relaxation to occur at its own pace. When distracting thoughts occur, try to ignore them by not dwelling upon them and return to repeating "one."
With practice, the response should come with little

effort.
Practice the technique once or twice daily, but not within two hours after any meal, since the digestive processes seems to interfere with the elicitation of the Relaxation Response.

* or any soothing, a mellifluous sound, preferably with no meaning or association, to avoid stimulation of unnecessary thoughts.

## Invite pleasure as your guide - learning to receive from the Universe

"If you change the way you look at things, the things you look at change."
— Wayne Dyer

You have the power to change your experience of stress by promoting pleasure in all areas of your life. By choosing to focus on positive, high-frequency places, people, and things, you will begin to notice dramatic shifts in your state of mind. Repeating a simple mantra such as, "I am good, healthy, vibrant and fertile," works on the deepest cellular levels to change the structure of how you feel, internally and externally. Physiologically, eliciting feelings of joy and pleasure cause the body to release a chemical called nitric oxide into the bloodstream. The more pleasurable the thoughts and experiences are that you flood your body with, the more the nitric oxide increases "feel good" chemicals in the body, including serotonin and beta-endorphins. This is most obviously experienced during an orgasm in both men and women. The act of becoming aroused immediately sends blood flow toward the genitals. Researchers have found that penile nerves produce nitric oxide: the chemical messages that allow an erection. Nitric oxide causes the blood vessels to relax. They then become filled with blood, and the erection occurs. Women have a central compass for pleasure in the clitoris, which has 8000 nerve endings dedicated solely to pleasure. [ix] Much like the relaxation response, finding multiple ways to release nitric oxide into your blood stream reduces stress chemicals like cortisol, and improves functioning in the parasympathetic nervous system. Becoming pregnant is a state of receptivity. Learning to receive pleasure is often one of the most important steps a couple can take to restore fertility.

Simply put, when we are moving in line with our highest good, we experience pleasure. While certain events and experiences can take cause us to lose this expansive feeling momentarily, we can make the choice each day to maximize pleasure in our lives. To prove the "pleasure principle", Health Scientist Dr. Deborah Kern tallied the results of a one-month study where 108 women focused on pleasure in their lives.[x] Kern coined the study the Pleasure Diet and her goal was to find women who spent most of their lives taking care of everyone but themselves, and to see how introducing pleasure in their lives could change their experience of stress. By using the five senses, women were asked to find pleasure each day and report back on the results. Participants were also asked to practice daily meditation, which research has shown to increase "feel good" chemicals, including serotonin and beta-endorphins. The results were amazing. In all twenty-two areas Kern observed, participants reported significant improvements in satisfaction levels, from their sex lives to sleep quality to health and careers, simply by adding pleasure into their lives.

To practice Kern's Pleasure Diet in your own life, she suggests starting by calling upon your five senses to reveal pleasures in your everyday life:

1. **Taste:** What appeals to your palette? Sour? Sweet? Salty? Savory? What are your favorite treats? A piece of high quality dark chocolate?
2. **Touch:** What feels good against your skin? Cashmere? Your partner's caress? A luscious bubble bath?
3. **Smell:** Lighting candles and incense? A fresh baked apple pie? Herbal teas? Scented Oils?
4. **Sight:** What sites bring you pleasure on a daily basis? Art? Photos of friends and family? Pictures from your travels?
5. **Sound:** Music can be relaxing. What do you crave? Classical? The sound of a friend's

laughter? Chimes?

Include items from each category in your life each day to fill yourself with pleasure and nitric oxide. To learn more about Dr. Deb and her pleasure diet please visit http://drdebkern.com.

## A shift in perception from fear to love

Every thought we entertain has a direct impact on our biochemical make-up. While we may like to think of our brain and our bodies as separate and distinct entities, it is well known that most of our receptors reside in the "gut," and furthermore, that the electromagnetic field of the heart is hundreds of times more powerful than that of the brain. The conclusion: in a battle between intellect and emotions, your emotions will always win.

Oftentimes we view the diagnosis of infertility from an intellectual standpoint, based on numbers that indicate imbalances in hormones, thickness of the uterine lining, and so on. What's less often recognized is that these intellectual numbers have a way of indicating whether we are doing "good" or "bad." How do we perceive ourselves and begin to "rate" ourselves in accordance with these numbers? What do these numbers actually mean? Some would argue that your chances of conceiving are far less dependent on your FSH score, and that your fertility outcome is far more dependent on the balance between your body, mind and emotions. At CNY Fertility Center, numbers are simply indicators to highlight various options we might use to bring balance to your body. My friend and colleague Randine Lewis has seen women with FSH levels as high as 108 go on to conceive to the shock of many other doctors. [xi] What I know for sure is that miracles happen everyday. Many of our age old beliefs are limited and contracting. The nature of fertility is expansive. In order to find the place of receptivity and deep healing, each client's feelings and innermost needs must be addressed. This is the place where western medicine and complementary medicine can work together to produce beautiful results.

When we look to our emotions, there is a temptation to label them as negative or positive. At each polarity our cells experience differing physiological reactions in the form of expansion or contraction that are eloquently described below in Dr. Bruce Lipton's theories on cell growth and development:

> In humans, the extremes of the two polarities might appropriately be described as LOVE (+) and FEAR (-). Love fuels growth. In contrast, fear stunts growth. In fact, someone can literally be "scared to death." Perception of environmental threats suppresses a cell's growth activities and causes it to modify its cytoskeleton in adopting a

protection "posture." Suppressing growth mechanisms conserves valuable energy needed in exercising life-saving protection behaviors.

Adrenal hormones also reroute brain blood flow by constricting forebrain blood vessels and dilating hindbrain vessels. Fight or flight situations are more successfully handled using hindbrain-mediated reflex behaviors. Constriction of forebrain blood flow suppresses "logic" or "executive reasoning," since slower thinking responses ultimately jeopardize fight-flight reactions.[xii]

The energy of the universe is expansive. Love expands, fear contracts. A diagnosis of infertility often brings with it a deep contraction, as we are overwhelmed with a multitude of emotions from guilt to shock to shame. How can our bodies be acting against us? While it's natural to experience a wide range of emotions, I have found that it is far more beneficial for my clients to shift towards positive thinking. This does not mean ignoring your feelings, which are deeply important to feel and express, but rather finding a way to shift towards positivity and support your greatest experience of health and happiness.

Knowing that we are chemically wired to resort to intellectual thinking in times of stress indicates that it is even more important to get in touch with our emotions than we might have previously thought. Through close examination, we can oftentimes trip our own wires and shift instantly from fear to love. Our ability to change our perception is a learned behavior and, like anything else, must be practiced. By releasing the constriction in your own body, you allow yourself to open up to the unlimited possibilities available to you in this present moment. With this simple shift, you can begin to live your most fertile life.

Just look at the research of Dr. Masaru Emoto, a visionary Japanese scientist who helps us tangibly understand the relationships between our body and our emotions, as exhibited by the impacts of words on water formations.[xiii] Dr. Emoto has shown that the molecular structure of water, which makes up 70% of the human body, is deeply impacted by human vibrational energy, thoughts, words, ideas and music. Through photography, Emoto has documented the changing shapes of water into beautiful crystalline apparitions, as they are doused with love and blessings. His message about the possibilities within the human body is powerful: by shifting our thoughts and vibrations, we have the ability to heal and transform our own lives as well as the lives of those we come into contact with.

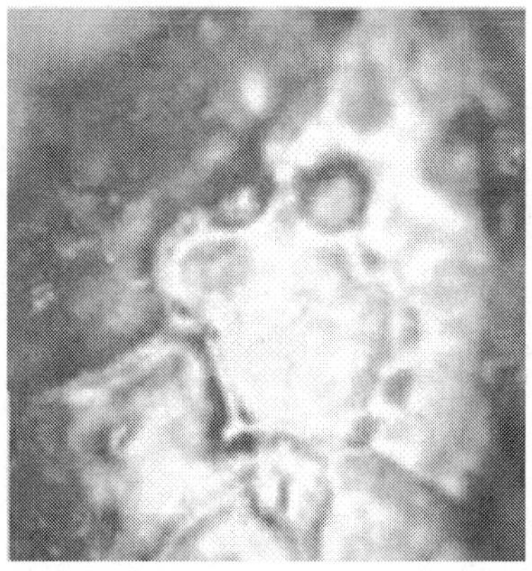

Image: Fujiwara Dam before offering a prayer

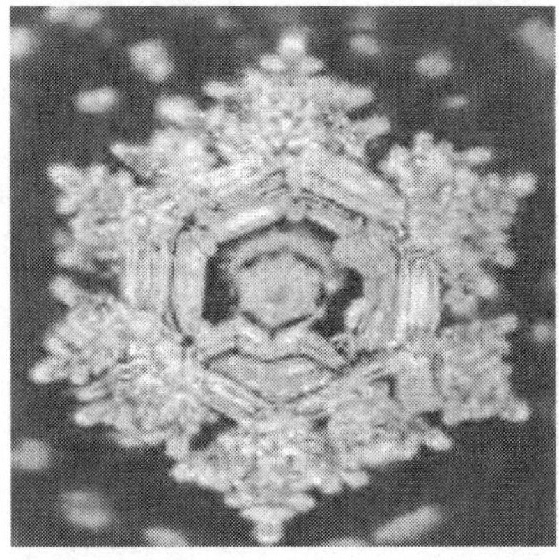

Image: Fujiwara Dam after offering a prayer

Not coincidentally, the element of water actually corresponds with reproductive function in Chinese medicine. According to eastern traditions the kidneys, adrenals and reproductive organs in both men and women all form together at birth. This triad contains our deepest essence or "Jing" which governs all developmental functions in our body, including fertility. Throughout our lives, we exchange our "essence" to live. When we overtax our bodies with stress, lack of sleep, poor nourishment and the emotion of fear, we deplete our reserves, which can manifest as challenges with reproduction.

**The Water Archetype:**

In the five-element theory of Traditional Chinese Medicine, the water element corresponds with a distinct personality that reminds us to nourish our deepest essence.

"She craves alone time. She is a philosopher who lives to reach the depths and discover life's truths. She has little time for small chat and yearns to know people at their core. Her idea of the perfect night is a good book and a bubble bath, safe from the chaotic outside world, yet she must balance her introverted nature, step outside of her comfort zone and share her insights and wisdom with the world. The power of water comes from the capacity to conceive, concentrate and conserve."[xiv]

Many of us live stressful lives, particularly in a day and age where we process more information in one day than our ancestors did in an entire lifetime.

Our nature is to be more outwardly focused, or "yang," and there is a tendency in the Western culture to reject our own internal needs, or "yin." The process of fertility involves accessing our deepest yin and replenishing our essence. To do this, we must become cognizant of the ways we are living our lives, and how stress and fear may be adversely impacting our ability to conceive.

Deep rest is the place of healing, so we must begin to look for areas in life that promote peace and wellbeing. For some, this may begin with simply getting adequate sleep, crucial for hormonal balance. According to a study from the University of Texas Health Science Center, "melatonin could become an important medication for improving ovarian function and oocyte [egg] quality."[xv] Melatonin is produced by our bodies in complete darkness and, therefore, those who stay up at night and sleep with lights on--or even turn lights on to go to the bathroom--are impacting their menstrual cycles and potentially missing out on the opportunity to improve ovarian function and egg quality. Create a sanctuary where you sleep: keep a clean, clear space where you can rest in complete darkness for 7-8 hours without external stimulation from light or electronics.

## Self-inquiry: Balancing action and replenishment

Yin vs. Yang: In the symbol below, brainstorm all of the activities that you do in a given day that would be considered an outward expenditure of energy (yang) vs. an inward accumulation of energy (yin).

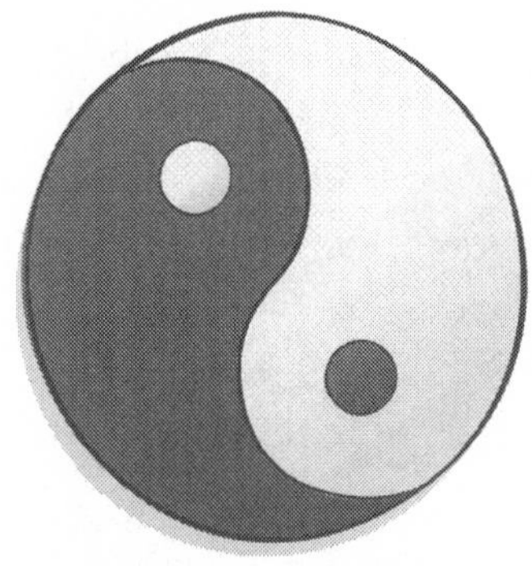

## The power of meditation

"When you are calm, you feel the whole universe of happiness rocking gently beneath your consciousness."
— Paramahansa Yogananda

Meditation is a powerful tool to train the mind to find peace and serenity, no matter what is happening around us. As the famous parable goes, The Zen master Nan-in received a visit from a university professor and offered him tea. When the tea reached the top of the cup, Nan-in just kept on pouring so that it spilled all over the table.

"Stop! Stop!" cried the professor. "It's too full!" "And you," said Nan-in, "are too full of your own opinions. How can you learn Zen like that? Empty your cup!"

Similarly, it easy for us to be filled to the brim with thoughts of what we need to do, should do, and can do for our fertility. Meditation is an essential practice for eliciting the relaxation response, which allows us to be receptive to the things we yearn for in our lives. In a revealing 1993 study, 4000 meditators were gathered from 81 countries in Washington DC with the intent of reducing the crime rate by 20% over an 8 week period.[xvi] With odds of less than 2 in one billion of other factors impacting the crime rates, researchers saw a 23% reduction in the area's crime rate. They concluded that meditation "creates a state of deep relaxation and coherence in the individual and simultaneously appears to produce an effect that spreads into the environment, influencing people who are not practicing the techniques and who have no knowledge of the experiments themselves."[xvii]

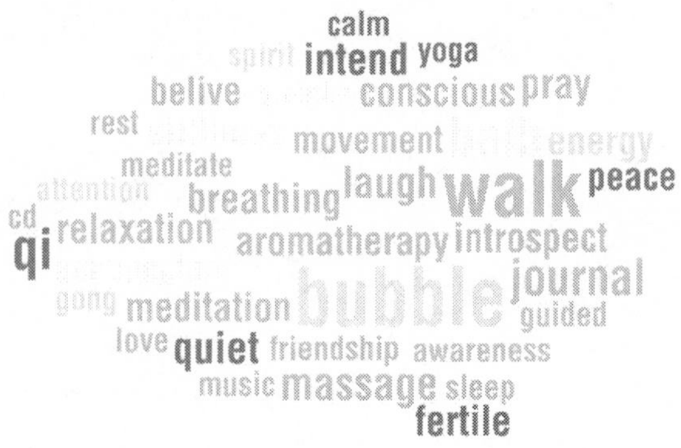


Instead of looking at meditation in the traditional sense, which can be overwhelming for beginners, start to imagine the variety of ways that we can spend just 12 minutes a day dropping into our inner experience for deep reflection to calm the mind, regenerate, and connect with our inner peace.

## 12 minute meditation using the power of visualization

"One reason we can change our brains simply by imagining is that, from a neuro-scientific point of view, imagining an act and doing it are not as different as they sound. When people close their eyes and visualize a simple object such as a letter a, the primary visual cortex is lit up, just as it would if the subjects were actually looking at the letter a. Brain scans show that in action and imagination, many of the same parts of the brain are activated. That is why visualization can

improve performance." [xviii]
— Norman Doidge

**Mapping Your Dream Garden**: an exercise to develop vision and intention using the law of attraction.

What you'll need:

- Old magazines
- A large Bristol board
- A glue stick
- A quiet space

Using visualization as a tool for manifestation can bring you closer to living your "best life". Your intention is powerful and will be used to bring you closer to your dream garden. Begin this exercise by entering into a quiet space and meditating for twelve minutes on "your best life." Close your eyes and breathe gently in and out, through the nose, focusing on your heart. What areas of your garden need cultivation? How can you nourish your body, mind and spirit? What would you like to draw into your life? Let your mind gently sift through the images and words that appear, noticing what brings you joy. Feel resonance in your heart as you imagine yourself living the life of your dreams. When you are ready open your eyes, begin looking through your magazines, tearing out images and words that symbolize that which you desire. When you feel complete, create the collage of your dream garden. Place your vision board somewhere you pass by frequently to serve as a reminder of all the goodness you want to draw into your life.

# Step 2:
# Shift from the Mind to the Heart

"A major contributor to the genesis of many diseases…is an overload of stress induced by unconscious beliefs. If we would heal, it is essential to begin the painfully incremental task of reversing the biology of belief we adopted very early in life. Whatever external treatment is administered, the healing agent lies within. The internal milieu must be changed. To find health, and to know it fully, necessitates a quest, a journey to the center of our own biology of belief. That means rethinking and recognizing--- re-cognizing: literally, to "know again"--- our lives." [xix]
— Gabor Mate

Though we have within us more neurotransmitters in the gut than the brain, we are a mind-centered culture that favors educated, rational decisions. From a very young age, we are trained to use our minds to analyze situations and determine risk versus reward prior to making a decision. Very few of us are taught to pay attention to the feeling deep within our gut that urges us to listen to our intuition.

When dealing with infertility, there is a certain amount of information that can be processed with the traditional definition of the mind. However, intuitive reasoning must also be relied upon to ensure that the choice is a heart-centered one. Stress tends to trigger left-brain thinking, which specializes in analyzing, logical thought, science and math at the expense of right-brain thinking, which governs intuition, creativity, art, music and feelings of connection. When you take a culture already trained to predominantly use left-brain functioning and add a stressful event like infertility, our body literally pumps cortisol, shifts into survival mode, and moves into "black and white" thinking, losing the insight gained by creative reasoning, which considers the bigger picture. Living solely from the left-brain resembles a mathematical equation. If I do this + this = my outcome is determined. When life throws us loopholes, it helps to call upon our right brain and begin to open to new ways of thinking and understanding our world.

**EXPERIENCE =**

**USABILITY / ANALYTIC + DESIGN / CREATIVE**

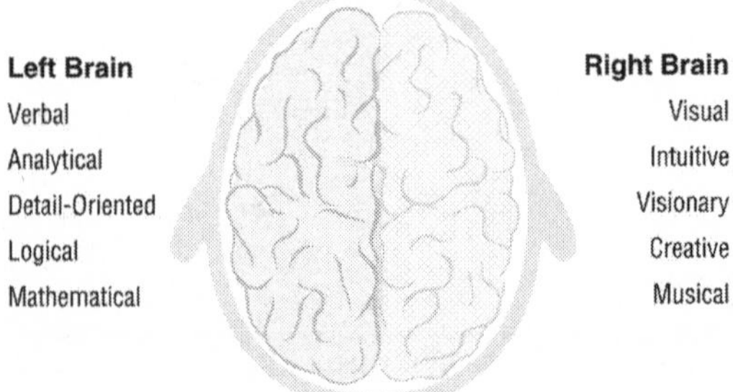

In the book, *Stroke of Insight*, brain scientist Jill Bolton Taylor explains how her own stroke allowed her to understand the role of the right and left-brain in determining reality. As she explains in her famous presentation at TED, the two hemispheres of our brain are completely separate with very distinct personalities.[xx] Our right hemisphere is about this present moment and thinks in pictures. Jill contends that the right brain gathers information from the energy all around us and gives us a picture of our present moment, through our senses, in the form of a collage. The left hemisphere thinks in linear terms and is focused on what we have learned in the past and how these lessons will determine our future. In the process of her stroke, she lost her left hemisphere function and experienced what she describes as true union with the universe, where all the stressors and emotional baggage that connect us to the outer world disappeared. Jill's stroke did for her what the diagnosis of infertility does for many, it provides a chance to slow down and look at life through a completely different lens. Though both diagnoses are clearly undesired, it is often only after the event that we can reflect and see the good that comes from challenging circumstances, the true gift.

What we know to be true is that our perspective can impact our outcomes. One study revealed that women who believed they would develop heart disease were four times more likely to, indicating that "if you believe something bad is going to happen, it probably will."[xxi] Considering the power of our thoughts alongside the fact that most of the 60,000 thoughts we entertain each day are repeats from the days before, it is worth it to stop in our tracks and examine whether our thoughts and feelings are in line with our desires.[xxii] When we fall into the habitual thought patterns of our left-brain, as Jill describes, we begin to determine our futures based on the information of our past, and often feel challenged to shift into right brain thinking. Although it may be challenging, the power lies within each of us to create the life we want. What we also know to be true is that "this coherency is at least partly within our control. Studies have shown that holding positive thoughts in our hearts creates coherency between electromagnetic and biophoton emissions, which then changes the DNA so that our bodies are healthier. In other words, DNA can at least partly be controlled by thoughts." [xxiii]

"Realize that your thoughts are real:

- You have a thought
- Your brain releases chemicals
- An electrical transmission goes across your brain
- You become aware of what you're thinking

Thoughts are real and they have an impact on how you feel and how you behave." [xxiv]

By visualizing the outcome we desire, we begin to create the blueprint for what can unfold. In moments when life is not what we believe it should be, perhaps it is an opportunity to use our imagination and begin to determine how the future will unfold. Look to the dream map for inspiration and relate to Mother Theresa's advice below. We must learn to focus on what we really desire for ourselves, rather than fight against the "problem we are experiencing": in this case, wellbeing in our bodies.

"I was once asked why I don't participate in anti-war demonstrations. I said that I will never do that, but as soon as you have a pro-peace rally, I'll be there." [xxv]

**Dr. Rob's Simple Strategies for Living Your Best Life:**

"You are a magnet attracting to you all things, via the signal you are emitting through your thoughts and feelings. To open yourself up and become a powerful magnet to wellness and health from wherever you are now:"[xxvi]

1. Go with the flow. The nature of the universe is change. Enjoy every step of the adventure.
2. Set your intention for healing. Hold thoughts of that which you want to create. The universe

is co-creating with your thoughts and feelings. Visualize yourself as you wish to be.

3. Laugh! It's contagious and does wonders for your health and the health of those around you.
4. One step further: give and receive a hug at least once a day. Touch is healing, and the positive vibration creates connection.
5. Look at your day with excitement and wonder. Being curious makes the mystery of life even more enjoyable.
6. Spread love and kindness everywhere you go. A simple smile or gesture goes a long way to changing the world.
7. Trade resentment for forgiveness. Learn to let go and shift to seeing the good in every situation instantly.
8. Express gratitude daily. Focusing on all that we have to give thanks for instantly shifts our vibration to receptivity.
9. See yourself fully fertile and vibrant: whole, healthy and powerful to create the life you desire.

The movie, The Secret, revealed just how powerful our thoughts are, and how becoming aware of the feelings that fuel our thoughts can help to create the outcomes we desire. The basic concept of the law of attraction is: like attracts like. What you are thinking and feeling is what you are seeing manifested in your life. There is a line in the movie that states: "You can have, do or be anything you want." [xxvii] The trick is to retrain the mind to focus on what you want rather than what you do not want. Many of us begin this process feeling somewhat disconnected from our thoughts and feelings. The first step is generally to stop and take notice of the tape that is playing in your mind without judgment. It is amazing the things we repeat in our minds without ever stopping to question: "I can't", "I should", "I'll never", and "I'm not good enough." Some of us exist with so many negative thought patterns that that we feel paralyzed. Locked up with thoughts about what we are not and what we can't be, we infuse our molecules with restrictions and as a result we end up dissatisfied with what we have. We limit ourselves with thoughts and labels without ever stopping to pose the question: "Is this true?"

Byron Katie, author of *Loving What Is*, and other bestselling books, travels across the country helping people to question their thoughts and end their suffering through a process she has developed called "The Work". Katie herself experienced severe depression and constant thoughts of suicide for ten years. Her turning point came with the following realization:

"I discovered that when I believed my thoughts, I suffered, but that when I didn't believe them, I didn't suffer, and that this is true for every human being. Freedom is as simple as that. I found that suffering is optional. I found a joy within me that has never disappeared, not for a single moment. That joy is in everyone, always." [xxviii]

Katie uses a three-step process that guides us out of catastrophic thinking by writing down the stressful thoughts that are making us miserable, investigating these thoughts, and experiencing their opposites. In the case of fertility it might be "I'll never have a baby," "I waited too long," "I shouldn't have spent so much time building my career," "It's my husband's fault that we waited." When you have written down your judgments, you then move forward through a self-inquiry process of four questions:

- Is it true?
- Can you absolutely know that it's true?
- How do you react, what happens, when you believe that thought?
- Who would you be without the thought?

Her third step is to turn the initial statement around by finding one or several opposites, and then find at least three genuine, specific examples of how these opposites are true in our life. In this process we come to notice that all our frustrations are merely projections and reflect our desire to control the world around us. Once we come to terms with radical acceptance of what is, we gain the freedom to choose where we place our energy. To experience the full process, please go to *http://www.thework.com* and download Byron Katie's process and handouts, available for free.

Sometimes simply facing our thoughts directly and questioning them allows for a shift in our thinking and serves as an "anteater" that helps us to overcome our internal "ANTS" or "automatic negative thoughts", a concept coined by Dr. Daniel G. Amen in his groundbreaking book, *Change Your Brain, Change Your Life*. Processes, like Byron Katie's, provide us with a reprieve from the day-to-day autopilot and give us the opportunity to place our thoughts back on our true desires.

The important piece is to question your thoughts without negating present moment feelings. When we are disconnected from our emotions or looking for ways to numb our pain, self-inquiry may bring painful emotions to the surface. No feeling is bad in and of itself. Many of us have grown up being taught to repress our emotions and to be polite, proper or good. In these instances, taking a closer look at what lies beneath the surface may feel more comfortable while working alongside a trained counselor. This helper acts as a compassionate witness to your experience as you release unconscious emotions that may be driving your thoughts.

Let us examine the role of the brain and the energy behind certain emotions to find ways to release automatic negative thoughts and move into positive creation. As we look deeper into some of our thoughts, you will begin to discern between those thoughts that are weakening and thoughts that are strengthening. When you allow yourself to fully feel where you are, you can begin the process of releasing what no longer serves you. Stuck emotions that may be holding you back on your fertility journey will give way to unlimited creative potential that will enhance your ability to use the law of attraction to create the life you desire. Remember to be kind with yourself throughout the process and continue to challenge your negative thoughts toward yourself, your life situation, and the world around you. As Wayne Dyer points out in his book, *The Power of Intention*:

"Low energy thoughts that weaken us fall in the realm of shame, hatred, judgment, and fear. Each of these inner thoughts weakens us and inhibits us from attracting into our lives what we desire. If we become what we think about, and what we think about is what's wrong with the world, and how angry and ashamed and fearful we are, it stands to reason that we'll act on those unkind thoughts and become what we're thinking about. When you think, feel, and act kindly, you give yourself the opportunity to be like the power of intention. While you're thinking and acting otherwise, you've left the field of intention, and you've assured yourself of feeling cheated by the all-creative Spirit of intent." [xxix]

As you delve deeper into this work and begin to

shake your old patterns for the sake of positive thinking and manifestation, you may come upon what Gay Hendricks describes in *The Big Leap* as the "Upper Limit Problem."[xxx] Basically we are used to only a certain level of success, happiness or pleasure. We will sabotage ourselves to get back to what is most comfortable. Watch for your own experience of the Upper Limit Problem as we move forward in releasing "weakening" emotions, thoughts and feelings in exchange for "strengthening" feelings. Our moods are, after all, the directors of our thoughts, emotions and experiences. Remember the power of visualization and begin to see yourself where you want to be. We have all heard the terms "acting as if" and "fake it until you make it." The process of imagining ourselves, as we would like to be is often part of the process that brings us closer to manifesting our desires.

"All negativity is caused by an accumulation of psychological time and denial of the present. Unease, anxiety, tension, stress, worry—all forms of fear—are caused by too much future, and not enough presence. Guilt, regret, resentment, grievances, sadness, bitterness, and all forms of non-forgiveness are caused by too much past, and not enough presence." [xxxi]
— Eckhart Tolle

## From fear and anxiety to a deep sense of security

"Being on the tightrope is living; everything else is waiting."
— Karl Wallenda

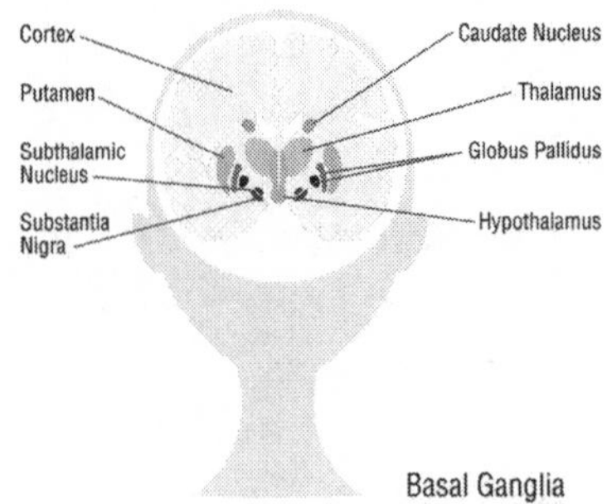


Basal Ganglia

The area of the brain that rules feelings of fear is the basal ganglia, (the area that surrounds the deep limbic system).[xxxii] This tiny area governs our primal reactions to the feelings we experience. For instance, when we feel someone coming up behind us, we get goose bumps. When someone startles us, we tremble. When the basal ganglia are ruling our lives, we are either paralyzed by fear, unable to act, or we are propelled into over-activity in an attempt to avoid the conflict and distract ourselves.

The truth is, so much of what we perceive to be stressful or are afraid of are events that have not--

and may never--occur. I often tell my clients that when the notion of fear arises, I have created an acronym to instantly shift my perception: **F**orget **E**verything **A**nd **R**elax. Fear is a primal feeling that was once associated with survival. When we would see a tiger, instinctually fear would motivate us to escape safely. Nowadays, the primal instinct that kept us safe on the plains of Africa is no longer necessary. Yet, we have adapted our survival mechanisms and fight-or-flight instinct to help us survive the concrete jungles of big cities and of our own minds. It is a fact that most of our deepest fears are imagined and self-created based on a future potential of threat. When we begin to face our fears directly, we acknowledge their existence and they immediately begin to dissipate. To calm the basal ganglia, we must call upon the wisdom of the relaxation response to remind ourselves that we are capable of dealing with what is put in front of us. Making time for quiet contemplation often brings us the wisdom to make a decision based on our present moment needs, as opposed to past events or future imaginings.

## 12 minute meditation to enhance peace

### Soak in Security

In Chinese Medicine, the emotion of fear is associated with kidney, adrenal, and reproductive function. In fact, animals in the wild do not reproduce when they feel the threat of danger. Just as in animals, the chronic state of stress that we experience can shut down secondary functions, including fertility, in an effort to preserve vital functions like our heartbeat. Today, practice shining the light of awareness on your perceptions of stress and fear. During your twelve-minute meditation, soak your feet in a warm footbath with sea salts. Water and salt are the corresponding elements to the emotion of fear and will help you feel grounded in safety and security.

## From anger and resentment to appreciation and gratitude

"We are so often caught up in our destination that we forget to appreciate the journey, especially the goodness of the people we meet on the way. Appreciation is a wonderful feeling; don't overlook it."
— Author unknown

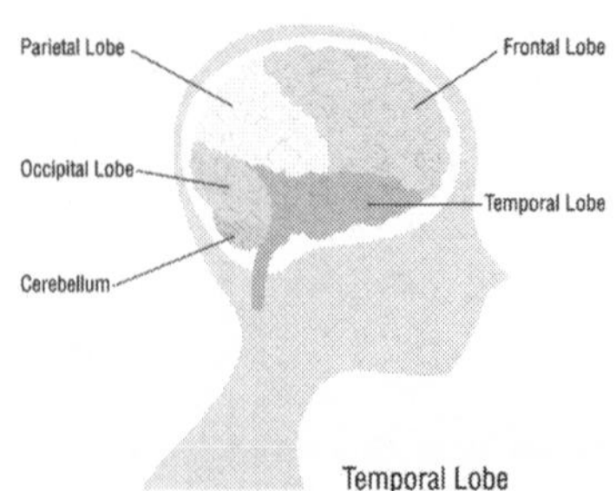

Temporal Lobe

The temporal lobe is the area in the brain where our memories are stored and our sense of self is developed.[xxxiii] The quality of our memories determines how we perceive the quality of our lives. In the case where someone has an abundance of happy memories, it is likely that they will experience the world through "rose colored glasses" with a good sense of self-esteem. In the case where the temporal lobe is storing many negative experiences, a person may exhibit deep sorrow and mood swings. Since this area of the brain is associated with past experiences, angers and resentments are not easily released until we move into the present moment and begin to recreate positive memories and associations. Positive thinking does not mean ignoring reality, it simply means finding ways that bring appreciation and gratitude into your life each day can impact the quality and perception of your life. Being happy does not mean everything is perfect; it means you have decided to look past the imperfections and focus on what you are grateful for.

Despite all the challenges we may deal with on a daily basis, there is no better gift to ourselves and others than the expression of love and appreciation for all that we have in our lives. This deep feeling of gratitude radiates through the universe and draws positive vibrations towards us. Scientific research at the Institute of HeartMath has shown that the respective feelings of resonance or dissonance impact our physiological wellbeing, perceptions, emotions and health. Knowing that a shift towards appreciation and gratitude can heal, let us consider how often we experience sentiments such as "I do not like," "I do not love," or even "I hate." By considering the unique gifts inherent in each person or situation, we can release negative energy and create space for positive vibrations. Today, practice shifting your energy towards resonance by expressing appreciation and gratitude at each opportunity.

## 12-minute meditation to enhance gratitude

### Resonating with the Heart

What you'll need:

- A private space (optional to play soothing music, which can soothe the temporal lobe, or have complete silence)
- HeartMath technology (optional)
- Ongoing: Keep a gratitude journal (see Kristen Magnacca's *Love and Infertility: Survival Strategies for Balancing Infertility, Marriage and Life*)

Shifting to a positive vibration requires nothing more than your willingness to experience appreciation and gratitude. Consider using the following exercise to shift towards positivity anytime you feel yourself falling prey to negative thoughts or energies. Begin by sitting comfortably and letting the eyes gently close. Focus on heart energy, breathing in and out through your nose. Sit quietly for the next twelve minutes or more, drawing in images of that which you love. You may initially choose the people that are closest to you and notice feelings of dissonance. This is a perfectly natural feeling as human relationships are dynamic, shifting from day to day, based on expectations. To induce a feeling of unconditional love, place your attention on a favorite pet or a place that brings positive, peaceful memories. When you feel a shift in your heart, stay with the feeling and enjoy the peacefulness that comes with resonance. Draw upon that image to bring to you to positivity and promote wellbeing in yourself and all those who surround you.

Note: If you feel you might benefit from additional support, the HeartMath Institute has a computer program that allows you to monitor your levels of resonance and dissonance and track your progress into the "green zone" of deep appreciation.

## From worry to acceptance

"If you change the way you look at things, the things you look at change."
— Wayne Dyer

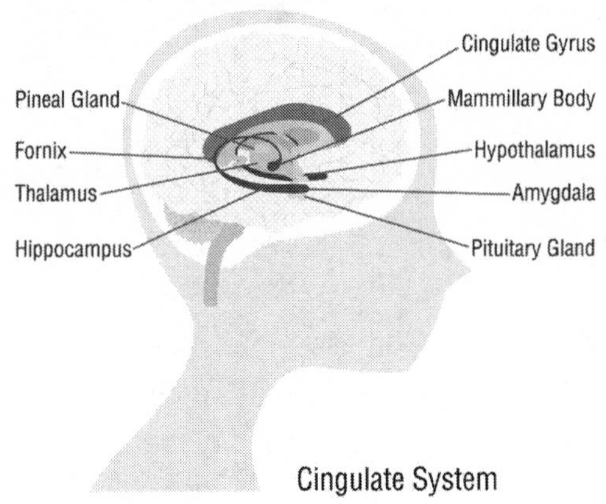


Cingulate System

The cingulate system in the brain governs our ability to adapt to change and transitions with a level of flexibility.[xxxiv] When the cingulate brain is not functioning properly, a person tends to predict the worst, is rigid in expectations and demands, and incapable of going with the flow or releasing grievances from the past. The health of this part of our mind thrives in a state of open consideration and acceptance of solutions that present themselves on our path.

It is certain that change is the one constant we can count on in life. For most, change often brings a level of uncertainty and discomfort. We often become comfortable in situations, even if familiarity is compromising our highest good. By learning to embrace change, we open ourselves to the unlimited potential present in our environment.

In fact, it is our resistance to change that can sometimes create obstacles to living our best life. Can you look back to a time where a perceived "bad" change brought you a hidden gift? Embrace change and learn to flow with life. When we are in the flow, we exist in our highest vibration and magnetize our desires to us.

## 12-minute meditation to enhance acceptance

The desire to keep things the same can contribute to a level of "stuckness." To maximize your creative potential and to be with the flow of life, institute change in your life today. Here are some ways to experience and learn to embrace change:

- Re-arrange your living space
- Paint your walls
- Color your hair
- Take a belly dancing class
- Donate clothes you haven't worn in 6 months
- Make a new friend
- Change your exercise routine
- Learn the serenity prayer: God grant me the serenity to accept the things I cannot change; courage to change the things I can; and wisdom to know the difference.

## From depression to positive experiences of self and others

"There is no remedy for love but to love more."
— Henry David Thoreau

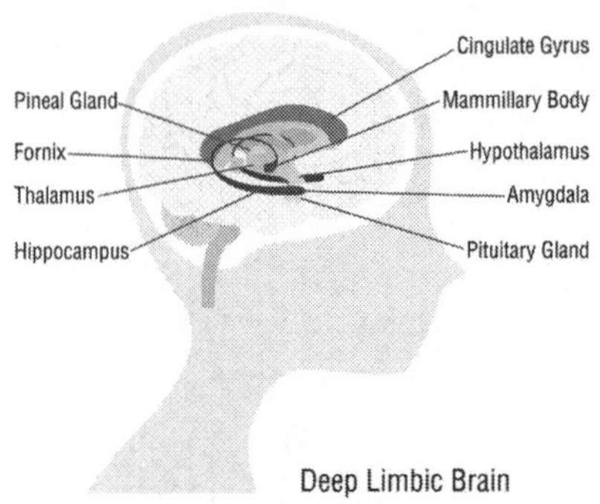


Deep Limbic Brain

The deep limbic brain is the area that impacts how we perceive our world and label events, people and situations as either good or bad.[xxxv] These labels determine the subsequent actions we will take, based on our perceptions. When we are depressed, there is a tendency to isolate and experience changes in appetite, sleep and motivation patterns. Stressful events, like challenges with fertility, commonly over-activate the deep limbic brain and cause problems in areas of bonding with partners, social connection, sexual function and sensory stimulation (think fresh roses or home-baked apple pie). Focusing on what we love can help to re-pattern this area of the brain.

Love is a single word that has so much meaning for all of us, yet is often easier to experience than to explain. According to many philosophers, the only goal of life is to be happy. And the only true happiness in life is to love and to be loved. In Greek culture, there are several different words to distinguish the various types of love. "Agape" translates to "I love you," the most common expression of true affection in our society. "Eros" expresses passionate love and sexual desire. "Philia" means friendship, and implies a deep loyalty towards one's tribe, friends and family. "Storge" is the affection used to describe the relationship between a parent and a child. Finally, "thelema" is a deep desire or longing to do something or be someone.

## 12 minute meditation to enhance positive perceptions

### Love All Ways Everyday

How many ways are you receiving love in your life? During your daily twelve-minute meditation, consider all the sources that you get love from and give love to. Feel love circulating through all of your cells and as you express gratitude for each type of love in your life.

After your meditation, use your gratitude journal and make a list to reflect upon all of the sources of love in your life.

Agape ______________________________

Eros ________________________________

Philia ______________________________

Storge ______________________________

Thelema ____________________________

**Understanding Grief on the Fertility Journey**
by Lisa Stack, CNY Fertility Support Coordinator

We often experience many moments of joy with the help of Dr. Rob and the rest of the CNY Fertility Family, whether it be in Syracuse, Rochester, or Albany. However, sometimes there are low moments of pain and grief. This is unfortunately natural in the world of fertility and creating families. Although we would love for the joy to stay, we unfortunately cannot control what happens. So what do we do when we experience a loss? We have to grieve.

The grieving process is different for everyone, and there isn't a set timeline or protocol to follow. It is extremely individualized and is completely dependent on the needs of those experiencing the pain. According to the Kübler-Ross model, there are typically 5 stages experienced during the grieving process:

1. **Denial:** This occurs with the initial shock of the situation. It may occur when you first hear 'I'm sorry but the test was negative' or when you first discover you need help creating your family. Naturally we will say to ourselves, or even out loud, 'No, it can't be,' or, 'I know you are wrong. Check again'. Our mind resorts to denial initially to protect ourselves from the reality of the situation. We find ourselves grasping for any sort of flaw in what we are being told, in order to prove to ourselves that it isn't true. Once the denial lifts and we begin to absorb what has happened, we tend to recognize our loss and the impact it will have on our lives. In the case of a miscarriage, you may begin to think of what the child's life would have been like, and the plans you had made for your family. This leads us to the next stage in grief: anger.

2. **Anger:** After denial of the situation and the beginning realization of the loss, it is common to feel angry. You might feel angry with yourself, with those around you, and quite often with God, or whatever spiritual being you associate yourself with. The anger comes when we realize our plans have been changed, and we will not have the life we

imagined before the loss. During this stage, it is common to feel angry towards those that are closest to you, even your spouse. You may feel they are not grieving properly or at all. This is OK. They may be in a different stage than you, or they may manifest their feelings differently. It is extremely important to realize that they are grieving, and that they are in pain. It is just not the same as yours. It is also important to note that men and women often experience a drastically different grieving process. After the anger subsides, it is common to begin the stage of bargaining.

3. **Bargaining:** Often bargaining occurs with the self, or with God. You may find yourself saying, 'Just let me have my child back,' or, 'Please just tell me what I can do to fix this situation.' Although we know we cannot change what has happened, this is another defense mechanism of the mind, body, and spirit: to make absolutely sure that there is no reversing the situation. This is similar to denial in that we are not ready to accept the loss.

4. **Depression:** During the fourth stage, depression, we begin to realize and acknowledge the loss. This is the most painful stage, and it can feel like it will never end. Often we can experience not just emotional and spiritual pain, but actual physical pain as well. This stage is the acknowledgement of the loss, and the recognition of the emptiness felt. It is often accompanied by

crying, feelings of abandonment, and wanting to withdraw from others. This is an incredibly important time of the grieving process, and it is not recommended to 'cheer the person up' or to try and distract them with other things. To truly mourn the loss, it is important to feel the depression, as difficult as that may be.

5. **Acceptance:** Once the depression lifts, you may feel a lift in your spirits as well. It is not that you have forgotten what has happened, or that you are any less upset about the loss. Instead, acceptance signifies that you have grieved, felt each step of the grieving process, and now you are looking for hope and a way to remember while moving on at the same time. Common ways to describe this stage are, 'I can't change what happened, I have to learn to live with it,' or, 'I will never forget, but I need to be able to live as well.' This is a time where you may want to be alone again, and that is OK. It can be difficult to navigate these new feelings of 'being OK.' You may feel guilty about trying to conceive again, or about taking some time for yourself. This is a stage of balancing grief, with life. While you may accept what happened and feel a little more comfortable about moving on with your life, it does not mean that you have forgotten, or that the pain will go away. You will still feel the pain of loss. However, it will not be as intense as it was in the beginning. You will be able to place it in better perspective now that you have accepted the situation.

While you are reading through the above stages, they may appear to make sense chronologically. However, remember that everyone grieves differently and in different stages. You may experience depression before anger, or you may skip a step completely. However it occurs is right for you. The important part is that you feel each step. As painful as it is, that is the only way to fully acknowledge and accept the loss you have experienced. You will also be able to mend the relationship with yourself, your spouse, family, and God (if this is appropriate,) while you grieve, because, unfortunately, relationships can suffer as well during a loss.

Perhaps the most challenging activity for the mind is the true experience of letting go. We are so used to judging ourselves for our thoughts and feelings that we perceive as negative that we become stuck. Self-forgiveness and self-acceptance are key ingredients to moving forward and living a life filled with kindness and compassion for yourself and others. Remember to focus on that which you desire. With alignment in your thoughts, feelings, and emotions, you can begin to create the life you want and use you inner strength to assist you on your healing journey. A new habit takes at least 21 days to groove in the mind, so be consistent with questioning your thoughts to retrain your brain.

**Week 16: Labels**
CNY Fertility client and blogger, April All Year

As I was climbing the long and winding staircase to the top of the lighthouse on our vacation, I thought about how we often become caught up in the labels we and/or others place on ourselves. For example, when I was first diagnosed with MS, I was terribly afraid I would lose my mobility, because that is the association I had with the disease. Here I was though, two years later, climbing to the top of Mt. Greylock's lighthouse, not succumbing to anyone's preconceived notions – not even my own. In fact, much of my thinking has slowly changed over the last several months.

I recently read the book, Inconceivable, by Julia Indichova, which chronicles this woman's journey beyond the labels she is given (high FSH, not IVF eligible). In the end, she achieves a miraculous pregnancy, because she does not allow herself to be restricted by the categories under which she falls. She refuses to succumb to anyone's preconceived notions.

Personally, I feel as though I surrendered to the label of "infertile" entirely too easily. Before the one-year point, I was nervous about not being pregnant, and had all of the fertility testing done. At the one-year point, I immediately began fertility treatment and moved through the range of options with little to no consideration of my own intuition, because I was already labeled as infertile. Thus, I simply did what the fertility center instructed me to do. When I took a break, I was tired of being told what to do, when to do it, and how to do it. I needed to reclaim some personal control over what often becomes an impersonal process.

As I did some research, I learned that I would not have already been classified as infertile in Europe, because they do not recommend fertility testing until the two-year anniversary of trying to conceive. If I were in Europe right now, I would just have finished my fertility testing, and would have only recently begun considering my treatment options. One of the lessons I have been slowly learning over the past year is that my own perception and intuition is far more important than any category I am placed in according to a statistic or by a physician.

Statistically, Julia Indichova had virtually no chance of achieving a healthy pregnancy. She was told to consider using donor eggs and/or a surrogate. Sometimes I become disheartened by the low statistics for pregnancy achievement for someone in my category (trying for more than two years), but then I remember that I am more than a statistic and that giving up simply is not an option.

I hope that we can each look deep within to see beyond the preconceived notions, so that we are able to truly tap into our intuition, find the strength from within, and move forward in the way that is right for each of us. Although a baby is miraculous, aren't our abilities to persevere and believe miraculous, too? My goal in the upcoming months is to forget the labels and trust that inner voice which I sometimes forget to recognize.

Miraculous blessings,
April all Year

# Step 3:
# Accept Support: Love and Infertility

From the day I began working with fertility clients, I recognized that infertility treatments were not something that could be tackled alone. When we face challenges in life, it is easy to become overwhelmed by the unknown and slip into anxiety and fear. It is during these moments that it is most important to learn how to nurture yourself and ask for the support you need. For each of us, this may mean something a little different. Sometimes fertility challenges can leave us feeling isolated among our closest family and friends. It is for this reason that I developed three programs to offer support along the fertility journey:

**Fertile Friends One-On-One Program:**
Fertile Friends pairs clients together based on their experiences with infertility. This program has been created, because many clients have said that friends and family who have been their support system for other life issues just can't compare to the understanding and support provided by another person who is going through the same struggle to conceive.

**Circle of Hope Peer Support Group:**
Circle of Hope is a peer support group for CNY Fertility clients who are having difficulty coping with the realities of infertility, pregnancy loss and treatments. This is an autonomous group that was created and run by former clients, and is a forum for clients to find support from others in the same situation. As a member of this group, you can ask questions about treatments, discuss how to emotionally cope with infertility, and learn about different paths to parenthood.

**Private One-On-One Support:**
If you are looking for a more private one-on-one support situation, there is a CNY Fertility Center Staff member who has been through the fertility journey experience herself. She offers her services as a lay support person and can be contacted through CNY Fertility.

Initially, when I started working with fertility clients, I noticed there was a lot of emphasis on fertility as a woman's problem. As a result, there was not enough support for the couple, whose relationship was deeply impacted by the infertility diagnosis. Fertility challenges can become financially, emotionally and physically stressful, impacting even the strongest of relationships. Our natural urge for physical touch and sexual union often becomes more goal-oriented at the risk of pleasure and spontaneity. We know that this occurrence is a natural physiological reaction, as stressful events can trigger a disconnection in the deep limbic system that governs bonding. It's important to recognize that there are steps you can take to restore this connection along the way. In *Change Your Brain, Change Your Life*, Dr. Amen offers five quick tips to support healthy limbic bonding: [xxxvi]

- **Be close:** physical proximity and closeness strengthen limbic bonding
- **Find compatible smells:** the limbic system is driven by pleasurable smells
- **Create a positive memory bank:** the more you focus on positive memories, the closer you will be
- **Touch often:** non-sexual and sexual touch support bonding, quelling the limbic system and helping to stabilize mood
- **Hold positive intention:** focus on the things you love about your partner each day

**Strengthening Your Relationship**
by Lisa Stack, CNY Fertility Support Coordinator

Throughout your journey to conceive, you may find a new strain on your relationship with your partner. This can be troubling, but it is extremely common, and there are things you can do to help get your relationship back on track.

The task I will be discussing today sounds too simple to be true: Have sex. Seriously! When was the last time you made love to your partner just for the fun, and the love of it? By now, you know exactly what day of your cycle it is, when you are ovulating, exactly what time you have to have sex because you took your Ovidrel last night and don't want to miss ovulation, and after sex you contort yourself into all sorts of positions with your legs up a wall or a mound of pillows underneath you. These are all great things for trying to conceive, but just do me one favor: Take a deep breath! Do you remember when you first met your partner? When you couldn't keep your hands off of each other, and loved each night you spent together, just the two of you? There is a reason for that: love! That is what brought you here, and why you want to have a child together so badly.

It is easy to get into a routine and forget the little things that make us so happy. How about tonight you just enjoy each other. Try to forget what day of your cycle it is, and how work was that morning. More importantly, remember why you are together, and why you care. You did not choose each other because of your prospective fertility. You chose each other because of many more, wonderful reasons.

Not feeling up for sex? Try a massage, or a nice bath, anything to get you two close, and feeling that love between you. Trust me, it will be a nice visit from the spouse you remember.

Creating space to nurture your connection with your partner is essential to your individual and collective wellbeing. A couple of years ago, I started to wonder what else we could offer our clients to bring support and help to enhance their relationships. As the universe always does, it provided me with the answer I was searching for. My brother, Ray, introduced me to his friend, Mark Magnacca, whose wife happened to be the award-winning author of *Love and Infertility*, Kristen Magnacca. Together we decided to make the work she created to support couples available to our fertility clients at CNY, with the ultimate goal of spreading the message of *Love and Infertility* globally.

## Love & Infertility

When trying to create a family, a couple's normal life can be immediately and radically changed. Feelings of confusion, hopelessness and loss of control can overwhelm couples working to over come their fertility challenges. The efforts to create a baby can override all.

The concepts shared through *Love & Infertility: Survival Strategies for Balancing Infertility, Marriage and Life* provide a lifeline for couples struggling with infertility. The book's overall theme first begins with love, loving yourself, and loving each other through the journey to fertility.

Offered here and in the book *Love & Infertility: Survival Strategies for Balancing Infertility, Marriage and Life* are two useful strategies and interactive exercises for men, women, and for both partners together: "The Honey-Do List Strategy" and suggestions to "Keep Time In Perspective".

Though this time of life may be emotional and strenuous, these insights can help you regain control of your life, your marriage and your happiness.

(The following two sections, The Honey Do List Strategy and Keeping Time in Perspective have been adapted from *Love & Infertility: Survival Strategies for Balancing Infertility, Marriage and Life* by Kristen Magnacca)

## The Honey Do List Strategy[xxxvii]

The rolling motion of the boat was not as debilitating as I thought it would be. We had been on this cruise for two days, and I felt as though I finally had my sea legs under me. Among the list of activities we had chosen for the day was skeet shooting off the back of the ocean liner.

Scanning the people standing in line, I noticed I was the only woman waiting for a turn at shooting the clay disk. The sailor in charge of loading the rifle and releasing the clay pigeons got a little annoyed when it was my turn.

"Have you ever shot a rifle before?"

"Nope," I replied.

His attitude was not what was advertised in the cruise brochure. He roughly positioned the rifle onto my shoulder and placed my fingers in the appropriate spots.

The weight of the rifle was more than I anticipated; my left hand drifted downward from the full weight of the barrel. I called out, "Pull!" and, forcing the rifle upward, I followed the clay disk with the nose of the barrel and shot the gun. I missed the target and was propelled backwards from the recoil. The impact of the butt of the rifle on my shoulder smarted more than I'd thought it would, but I motioned to the sailor to release another disk. By the end of my third try at shooting, I had gotten the hang of it—the stance, the balance of the gun, and the bracing for the recoil.

That night, back in our cabin, I noticed Mark leaning over the daily activity sheet that had been placed in our room the night before.

"The midnight buffet—check; daily run—check; skeet shooting—check;" he said as he crossed off the words on the list.

"My shoulder can attest to that!" It bore the brunt of my stubbornness and was turning an interesting shade of black and blue.

"Conga line—check; daily excursion—check. All done." Mark reached for a folder bearing the cruise line's emblem and carefully slipped the sheet inside it. As I watched him, I noticed two other sheets in there, already checked and placed there for safekeeping.

Closing the covers, Mark glanced my way. "All done?" I asked.

"Hey, I think I'm doing good being disconnected from work. I just need to feel that sense of accomplishment."

For some reason, Mark's habit of checking off his daily activities stuck with me. We used this strategy on weekends to motivate him to focus on what needed to be done around the house. Together, we would write a list and take a break after each task to check it off. It goes back to the fact that Mark moves toward pleasure, and he got pleasure from watching his list dwindle down to nothing. He needed to see what was done and what needed to be completed.

Three years into our attempts at creating our family, our marriage was just as bruised as my shoulder had been from the rifle—from the time it took to uncover the physical issues impeding our attempts to get pregnant, our failed two intrauterine insemination attempts, and then the joy of hearing that we were successful crushed when I was rushed to the hospital for emergency surgery that resulted in the loss of our baby and damage to one of my fallopian tubes. But in the case of our marriage, the cause of the bruising was invisible. It was the pure emotional trauma that we both attacked so differently while trying in vain to help the other person. We had sought out professionals to help us navigate the unknown territory of infertility, we asked for guidance from our doctors, we went to marriage counseling, and still we were drifting apart like the dividing wake behind our beloved cruise ship.

Logically, I knew that every marriage had its own flow and cycle, and when the flow of energy is compromised by stressors—such as getting a new house or a new job, attempting to have a child, or dealing with a miscarriage—these life events change how you communicate and view yourself, your partner, and your marriage.

We both realized that we were in conflict, and we were trying in vain to fix the problem. To make matters worse, in the midst of it all we weren't communicating, we weren't participating in each other's day. We lived in the same house and mourned our circumstances separately.

One morning, I woke up and realized that the pregnancy we had lost might not be the only tragedy that we could encounter, that our marriage was teetering dangerously close to falling overboard without a life preserver. I knew I had to do something. I wanted to get back to the point where we both felt good about our partnership. Remembering how we used to talk about everything and anything, and how that made everything feel so real, I desperately wanted that feeling back. Then I asked myself, what did Mark do that made me feel loved, appreciated, and secure?

The answer came back to me in images. Our first date popped into my mind: We had talked the night away. The images fast-forwarded through our numerous dinners, which included talking, talking, and more talking. Next, I thought back to our old nightly routine of going to bed together, reading and sharing with each other the words on the pages in our hands. These images and memories freshly in mind, I pulled out a stack of colored 3x5 cards from my office, and picked a bright pink card off the top. On the top line in the left-hand corner, I started to number the lines. Then I wrote down the three things I needed from Mark that day. I was hopeful that they would bring back the lost feeling of connection we'd had:

- Call me three times today
- Have dinner with me
- Go to bed with me and read

There it was. That was what I needed, three things from Mark, and they all boiled down to being together: physically together, sharing again, the normal relationship things. On the back of the card I wrote a line from our wedding vows: "Through sickness and health, in good times and bad. June 10, 1995."

The next step was to sell this to Mark. I greeted him with coffee and the bright pink card. At first, as usual, he gave me a blank stare as I explained how I thought this would work. Each morning, we could exchange cards with three things we needed from each other that day, and at the end of the day, we could hand back the checked- off card. And, if we felt like it, we could write a quote on the back. It was something we both could do that would give us a sense of fixing what wasn't working.

Mark still looked a little dazed, but then it was his turn to write down what he needed. On his first card he wrote the following:

- A proper greeting when I get home
- Remind me why you married me
- Ask me about my day and listen with

interest

It was all so doable! I knew the proper greeting was important for Mark, and I withheld it because I knew it bothered him! Remembering why I married him was easy, and to listen was what I longed for, too, but my bitterness had taken away any generosity of spirit I might have had to be the first person to break the ice.

It was amazing how this piece of paper changed our energy toward our marriage. Instead of indifference, we had connection. It got to the point that we were surprising each other with cards in unusual places—taped on the fridge, pinned to the shower, and in our giddiness we took our requests to the extreme.

One night, as he was driving up the hill to our house, Mark decided to fulfill his third call of the day to me and called me from his cell phone.

"I'm coming home to you, baby," he said. I could feel his mood shift from not wanting to come home, to anticipating us being together.

"Yippee!" I opened the door and ran to our driveway to wait for his car.

As he turned the corner into our driveway, I proceeded to jump up and down and scream, "You're home, you're home!" Now, that was a proper greeting! He was very embarrassed and, although he didn't admit it, flattered.

That night after dinner, while handing me back my lime-colored index card, Mark smiled and said, "I feel like a great husband."

"You know what, baby? You are!" And we locked each other in a tight hug.

I look back at how we struggled to find someone or something to help us communicate and cope with all that had happened to us on the journey to create a family, and it came down to communicating what we needed and not withholding what the other needed. We'd been playing "mind-reader," assuming that the other person should know what we wanted or needed without having to say it out loud. Then we'd become resentful when the other person wasn't fulfilling our needs. I felt that Mark already knew what I needed, but wasn't taking steps to help me. I certainly didn't know what Mark needed, and he wasn't telling me. The Honey-Do List strategy was a clear-cut way of getting our needs met and communicating them in a non- threatening manner.

We started using this strategy four years ago. We exchanged cards daily for three months, then, when we felt as though we had integrated each other's needs into our daily lives, we moved away from this strategy for a short period. When Mark's schedule required him to be away for days at a time, we would write out the appropriate number of cards and keep up the Honey-Do List even though we were miles apart. Continuing to use this strategy even when we were miles apart kept the momentum going and kept us connected during the separation.

Now we use our 3x5 cards as a fallback strategy to cut short marital misunderstandings or when one of us is feeling unappreciated, unloved, or misunderstood. I saved our cards in a filing box and sometimes pull out Mark's old cards and remind myself what it takes for me to meet his needs.

**Putting it into practice:** Pick up a packet or two of 3x5 index cards. We think the brightly colored ones are fun, but of course that's up to you.

**The basic rules are straightforward:** Every morning, each partner dates a card and writes three things that he or she needs from the other person that day. On the back of the card you can write a quote or a saying that you feel is appropriate. Then exchange your cards.

**Have some fun with this:** Try hiding the cards around the house, putting one on your partner's dashboard, slipping another into a briefcase (make sure it's easy to find).

During the day, as you fulfill your partner's needs, check them off the list.

At the end of the day, return the checked-off card to your partner. If for some reason a request hasn't been completed, then that person is responsible for explaining why and requesting another day to fulfill that obligation.

This strategy truly helped save our marriage. And other couples have found success with it, too. The day after Mark and I presented our Honey-Do List during a seminar, I received the following e-mail from a woman who was in the group. She wrote:

"With my 3x5 card in hand, I ventured off today feeling SO MUCH MORE connected to my husband than I have in months. Just by reading his first request, 'Wake me and say I love you BEFORE you go to work'...made me feel like he really DOES still care. Thank you and Mark for this, Kristen. We intend to keep this journey going with these cards, as we continue our infertility journey. It has been a long five years, and what you said last night really stuck. We both thank you most sincerely!"

Albert Einstein once said, "Everything should be made as simple as possible, but not one bit simpler." We should all take his lead and incorporate his philosophy into strengthening our relationships.

## Keep Time In Perspective[xxxviii]

My girlfriend sent me one of those annoying e-mails that, forward by forward, get passed around the world. The subject line, "Why Women's To-Do Lists Never End," was the only reason I opened the e-mail.

According to the story, even with a focused to-do list, a woman is left at the end of the day feeling as though she didn't get enough done. During the process of completing her required tasks, she inadvertently gets sidetracked by life.

The e-mail went something like this (I'm inserting my real life here):

She starts off down the stairs to put a glass in the dishwasher before leaving for work. When she arrives in the kitchen, she notices the table wasn't wiped. She wipes the table and brings the dishtowel to the laundry area where she puts the towel in the washing machine, which completes a full load, so she presses the start button. Heading back to the dishwasher, she notices her husband's nightly snack dishes left by his favorite chair. Picking them up to add to the dishwashing load, she stops and folds the blanket that should be on the back of the chair. Finally putting the glass and snack dishes in the dishwasher, she notices that the rinse agent light is glowing on the washing machine and stops to add that in.

Grabbing her coat to go to work, she sees that the trash hasn't been taken out and begins to sort the recyclable paper, plastic, glass, and tin into their appropriate bins. She carries the trash outside, gets into her car, takes a deep breath, and wonders why she's feeling behind already. Glancing down, she sees that the low-fuel light is on and, sigh, she's off to the gas station! While reaching for her credit card en route to the gas station, she notices that the purple dry cleaning bag on the passenger seat, placed there by her spouse, is now her morning companion for the ride to work. After wiping her hands off so as not to smell like gas, she decides to take the long way to her appointment so she can go through the drive-thru at the dry cleaners and ensure that the clothes will be ready in time for an upcoming business trip.

She arrives at the restaurant for her breakfast meeting just in time, requests to be seated, and waits a few seconds for her party to arrive. During those few moments she opens her day planner and reviews her daily to-do list. Number One stares back at her: Stop at the post office to mail work packets. Oh, man, she thinks, I'll swing there afterward. The meeting goes well; she assembles her meeting action items and feels confident that this relationship is a match. Jumping in her car, she dishwasher, she notices her husband's nightly snack dishes left by his favorite chair. Picking them up to add to the dishwashing load, she stops and folds the blanket that should be on the back of the chair. Finally putting the glass and snack dishes in the dishwasher, she notices that the rinse agent light is glowing on the washing machine and stops to add that in. Grabbing her coat to go to work, she sees that the trash hasn't been taken out and begins to sort the recyclable paper, plastic, glass, and tin into their appropriate bins. She carries the trash outside, gets into her car, takes a deep breath, and wonders why she's feeling behind already. Glancing down, she sees that the low-fuel light is on and, sigh, she's off to the gas station! While reaching for her credit card en route to the gas station, she notices that the purple dry cleaning bag on the passenger seat, placed there by her spouse, is now her morning companion for the ride to work. After wiping her hands off so as not to smell like gas, she decides to take the long way to her appointment so she can go through the drive-thru at the dry cleaners and ensure that the clothes will be ready in time for an upcoming business trip.

She arrives at the restaurant for her breakfast meeting just in time, requests to be seated, and waits a few seconds for her party to arrive. During those few moments she opens her day-runner and reviews her daily to-do list. Number One stares back at her: Stop at the post office to mail work packets. Oh, man, she thinks, I'll swing there afterward. The meeting goes well; she assembles her meeting action items and feels confident that this relationship is a match. Jumping in her car, she drives to the post office, mails the packages, and purchases stamps for an upcoming mailing.

She arrives at her desk in time for a conference call, which goes well, and then turns her attention to an urgent situation that has developed regarding an upcoming speaking event.

Her computer clock shows that it's after lunch; she'll eat later. She regroups to push ahead on her list of things to do. It's 2:30 in the afternoon, and only two things are crossed off.

Feeling a bit of tightness in her chest, she fills her glass of water and starts making her calls, completing only two of the four after being interrupted a few times to answer inbound calls. She reminds herself she has a meeting with the graphic designer at 4:00 PM and realizes if she leaves now, she'll be able to make it to the bank to make a deposit on the way. Taking a few minutes to organize herself for the 4:00 meeting, she grabs the appropriate folders and some UPS packages that need to be put into the box before 5:00 PM for next-day delivery. With her coat on one arm, she reaches for her to-do list and dates the next sheet in the pad for tomorrow, transcribing numbers four to six on tomorrow's list. Now she feels a bit inadequate. How could she only have finished three things today?

Running out the door while putting her coat on, she's back in the car and arrives at the UPS box, double-checks that the envelopes are securely in the box, jumps back in the car, and arrives on time for her meeting. She signs off on the design of the brochure, okay's the price for printing, and is off to the grocery store for dinner supplies.

Feeling tired and somewhat confused about how she so mismanaged her time that she didn't finish her to-do list for the day, she prepares dinner, does another load of laundry, and tidies up the house. Dragging a bit now, she heads upstairs to wash her face and put her pajamas on, but first she turns on the dishwasher, empties the laundry basket, refreshes the towels in the bathroom, reads her e-mails and responds to a few of them. At last she washes her face and climbs in bed, exhausted. She reaches for her journal and wonders how to start today's entry.

"I didn't really get that much done today..." she writes.

How far from the truth is that?

Yet how true it is for all of us, especially women. We are in constant motion—doing, doing, doing—and accomplishing so much each and every day that enhances our lives, yet we feel as though we haven't done enough. How accurate the subject line was of that e-mail; we are never truly done with our doing. And this applies to men as well as women. Time keeps on running, running, running, and it seems it's always running away from us and we never seem to catch up.

But what we must keep in mind, the really important part, is that in our doing we are also being. By being, I mean being who we are as people, being part of the process of creating—and that includes creating a family and also being aware of both.

**Putting it into practice:** How can you keep time in perspective? I believe that things happen for a reason and each of us is where we should be, doing exactly what we are supposed to be doing, at every moment in time. You can take the following measures and give yourself permission to be happy with the work you do.

**Recognize:** Tell yourself that you are in the process of creating your child, and you are right where you need to be today, doing exactly what you are supposed to be doing, and what you accomplish is enough. You've done enough.

**Reassess:** Just like when you are at work and, in the heat of doing what you are doing, you don't always notice your efforts, the same is true regarding the steps you are taking to make parenthood a reality. You might not think that you have done anything to move the ball closer to creating a family, but in reality you are! Have you eaten correctly? Yes! Taken your folic acid or vitamins? Yes! Your partner has on his boxers, correct? You're monitoring your cycle, and documenting the time of your ovulation, right? Of course you are! You've had blood tests and an ultrasound to assess your fertility cycle, right? All these are part of the process of creating and the concept of being in the moment. Appreciate yourself and your accomplishments.

**Remind:** Finally, remind yourself that what is consistent in any process is the beginning, middle, and the end, and as with all things, this process will come to an end. You're doing everything you can, starting at the beginning, working through the middle, and anticipating a positive ending.

# Step 4:
# Vibrate at Your Fertile Frequency

We are energetic beings that vibrate according to the pulse of our thoughts, interactions and environment. As a species, human beings are 99.99% genetically similar with a mere .01% difference in each of us that accounts for our unique attributes of look, personality, predisposition to health and ultimately how we respond to the world around us.[xxxix] Energetically speaking, health is resonance with that which is, while a lack of health can be seen as a state of dissonance. As Barbara Marx Hubbard alludes to in *Conscious Evolution*, a perceived state of dissonance--as in the case of challenges with fertility--may be offering us the opportunity to adapt.

"Let's compare our situation with the metamorphosis of a caterpillar into a butterfly. When the caterpillar weaves its cocoon, imaginal disks begin to appear. These disks embody the blueprint of the butterfly yet to come. Although the disks are a natural part of the caterpillar's evolution, its immune system recognizes them as foreign and tries to destroy them. As the disks mature and become imaginal cells, they form themselves into a new pattern, thus transforming the disintegrating body of the caterpillar's immune system breaks down and its body begins to disintegrate. When the disks mature and become imaginal cells, they form themselves into a new pattern, thus transforming the

disintegrating body of the caterpillar into the butterfly. The breakdown of the caterpillar's old system is essential for the breakthrough of the new butterfly. Yet, in reality the caterpillar neither dies nor disintegrates, for from the beginning its hidden purpose was to transform and be reborn as a butterfly." [xl]
— Barbara Marx Hubbard

Over years, the human species has evolved. While the goal of life was once to survive and reproduce, with the advancement of informational technologies and the bombardment of information, we as human beings have evolved beyond our basic needs. We have moved into a stage of co-creation where energy must flow freely and creative solutions are necessary to prevent stagnation. Our energies must be constantly re-attuned to vibrate in resonance with our environments and support health.

Our minds tend to prefer that which is quantifiable and measurable: what we recognize as Western Science. We now rely on tools to diagnose and measure our health, but before these "tests" existed, we had nothing to rely on but energy and intuition. As Western and Eastern medicines continue to merge, we are being reminded of what our ancestors have known for years: intuition and self-knowledge are sometimes more accurate than diagnostics. In one study, medical intuitive Carolyn Myss had a 90% accuracy rate when diagnosing medical conditions intuitively with only the client names and age compared to a 50-80% error rate in Western diagnostics."[xli] "To date over 150 controlled studies of healing have been published, with more than half revealing an effective application of intuition." [xlii] And yet, as a culture, we are still on the edge of accepting intuition as a valid form of diagnoses. We are so used to handing our health to a technician with the answers that we have lost the direct connection to the wisdom present in our own hearts. To regain connection with our intuition, understanding our own energetic system is helpful.

By definition, energy is that which fuels action. In it's truest form, energy is comprised of information that causes an impact on cells and atoms. Energy vibrates according to interaction and information. Consequently, we each have a profound impact on how our body responds, based on the messages we receive in our environments and through our thoughts and actions. Attuning your senses to perceive subtle energetic interactions within your body is an invaluable tool to diagnosing "problems" and imbalances before they occur. This allows for holistic medicine to interject and offer relief before the imbalance reveals itself on the surface and western medicine is needed.

Our most subtle energies (L-fields) combine with our thoughts (T-fields) to create resonance or dissonance within our bodies. Through technologies like HeartMath, the electromagnetic fields of the heart can now be measured and translated to infer how our frequency is impacting the cellular makeup of our bodies. HeartMath is a useful training tool to remind us how to return to a state of resonance and vibrate at our highest frequency. A highly resonating heart--like that of the Dalai Lama's--is believed to extend many miles in radius from his physical body. Of course, the Dalai Lama entrains his vibration daily through devotional practices like meditation, which can return us to the present moment and increase feelings of appreciation and gratitude, measurable by the HeartMath technology.[xliii]

If meditation can impact the crime rates of a major metropolitan city, it makes sense that shifting our personal vibration into a state of resonance could have a truly profound impact on our physical body. In much the same way as positive thoughts and vibrations bringing the body into alignment, our own limiting beliefs can lead to internal dissonance. Michael Jospe, a professor at the California School of Professional Psychology, refers to this dissonance as the "Nocebo effect" noting that, "If you believe something bad is going to happen, it probably will." [xliv] When we make the conscious choice to operate on a higher frequency, it is important to pay attention to our beliefs, continuously shifting our awareness to ensure our intention remains focused on greater health and enhancing our fertility. Equally important to our own beliefs is the orientation of the practitioners we are working with. Jospe has studied the effect of practitioners on their clients and has observed that, "The placebo effect is part of the human potential to react positively to a healer," and also that, "a healer's attitude helps create client outcomes." For what we do know is that, "the heart is 60 times more powerful than the brain [and] through this field, a person's nervous system tunes in to and responds to the magnetic fields produced by the hearts of other people." [xlv]

On top of our thoughts there has also been a shift in the magnetic field of our earth causing increased levels of geopathic stress. Our nervous systems rely on the magnetic field to recharge the entire system by helping the body deliver adequate nutrients to cells and organs. Over the past 4000 years, the magnetic field has diminished from 2-3 gaus to ½ gaus, leaving us less of a charge so to speak.[xlvi] This fact combined with the increasing electromagnetic pollution in the form of cell phones, x-ray machines, pesticides, hormones in our foods (xenoestrogens), and pollution, causes a direct impact on our health and wellbeing. Knowing that geopathic stress exists is not meant to create a culture of fear, but rather to instill the importance of taking pro-active steps to magnify health and wellbeing by making positive lifestyle choices that are within our control.

### What are xenoestrogens and where are they found?[xlvii]

Xenoestrogens are foreign estrogens that may interfere with our natural hormone pathways. There are nearly 70, 000 chemicals currently in use in the United States that are known to be toxic and impact hormones, specifically a condition known as estrogen dominance which can lead to reproductive disorders including low sperm count and fibroids. The National Institute of Environmental Health Sciences and Center for Disease Control and Prevention are in the process of studying 50 environmental estrogens to determine the impact of their toxicity on the human body. While our body is built to detoxify and release toxins, it is a good idea to avoid excessive chemicals where possible and cleanse through healthy lifestyle choices.

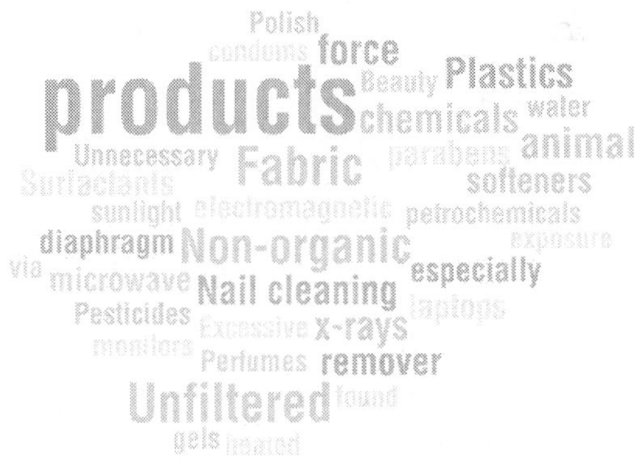

# Re-aligning your inner energy compass to attune your vibration

## The Chakra System "Energy Processing Centers"

Beyond the workings of our external body, we each have within us an internal compass comprised of seven chakra centers, which follow the path of the spine from the base to the crown of the head. The first chakra is located at the base of the spine, the second at the navel center, the third at the solar plexus, the fourth at the level of the heart, the fifth at the throat, the sixth between the eyebrows and the seventh at the top of the head. Chakras can be seen as energetic wheels, often pictured as lotus flowers that spin, acting as energy processors for internal and external messages, vibrating interpretations of resonance or dissonance to our nervous systems.

The chakras connect us with our inherent nature and both take in and send out energy. They are part of the electrical body, which is best restored when we reconnect with nature and often serve as indicators of whether we are living in balance or out of balance with our bodies. Much like the meridian system, the chakras allow energy to pass through freely when we are clear and balanced in the interconnection of our physical, subtle and emotional bodies.

The base of the chakra houses the kundalini energy, believed to be the seed of creation. In *Spirit Babies*, Walter Makichen describes the energetic conception chalice that creates the opportunity for a child to enter the body. The kundalini rises from the first chakra, sacral area, and spirals up through each chakra center up to the crown chakra where it opens into a bowl shape revealing the conception chalice:

"When couples with a conscious or unconscious desire to have a child make love, their kundalini energies flow up their spine and out the top of their heads. Their individual energies intertwine, forming a column. At the top, the two energies merge into the shape of a bowl. The whole form resembles a large gold and orange goblet or chalice. This gold and orange bowl, which I call the "conception cradle," floats above the top of the prospective mother's head. The conception cradle calls and welcomes the spirit baby, drawing the spirit into the conception contract. If the spirit baby enters the conception cradle, it begins to move down the mother's spine to her uterus. Safe in the conception cradle, the spirit crosses over from the spirit baby world and makes first contact with its new body. If the spirit baby accepts the new body, the fertilized egg will successfully plant itself in the mother's womb. The conception cradle then transforms itself into an energy cord connecting the spirit to its growing body. This cord is one of the foundations of human life. It allows the spirit's life force to animate and sustain the body. Formed at conception it is the last connection to be dissolved at the time of birth." xlviii

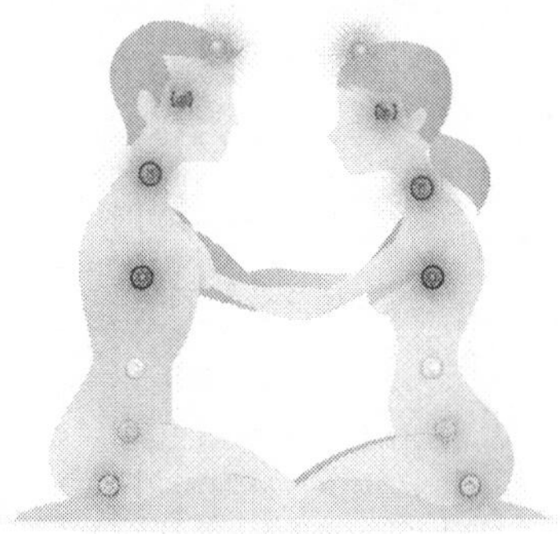

## Self-inquiry: Energy center resonance

In order for the kundalini energy to flow freely, it helps to understand the issues of each chakra system and work through any areas of blockage that can be freed up on the physical or emotional plane through self-inquiry. Though the second chakra (navel center) directly relates to reproductive function, a blockage at any level of the chakras may impact fertility. Self-inquiry into areas of blockage combined with meditation and visualization on the symbol, related color and intention can be helpful to clear energy flow and release kundalini.

**I AM (Muladhara)**

The First Chakra is located at the base of the spine, between the anus and genitals, and emits the color red. Known as the root chakra. This energy center rules our primal needs dealing with survival issues and feelings of security and grounding. When we are centered in the root chakra, we are supported in physical and psychological wellbeing. Related organs include the adrenals, bones and coccyx.

- Do I feel safe in my world?
- How are my energy levels?
- Am I focused or feeling scattered?

**I FEEL (Svadhisthana)**

The Second Chakra rests below the navel and emits the color orange. The sacral chakra governs our reproductive energies along with pleasure and creativity. Our emotions are the compass for navigating the feelings of this chakra. When the sacral chakra is open, sexuality, fertility and self-expression flow freely. Associated organs include sex organs, the bladder, the prostate and kidneys.

- Am I feeling vital and desiring?
- Do I have creative expression in my life?
- What brings me pleasure?

**I DO (Manipura)**

The Third Chakra sits above the navel and resonates with the color yellow. Known as the solar plexus, this chakra is the center of our personal power, will, and how we express ourselves in the world. When the third chakra is in alignment, we feel purposeful, productive and assertive with our emotions. Associated organs include the digestive system, the nervous system, and the immune system.

- Do I feel in control of my life?
- Does my occupation feel meaningful?
- Can I express my emotions clearly?

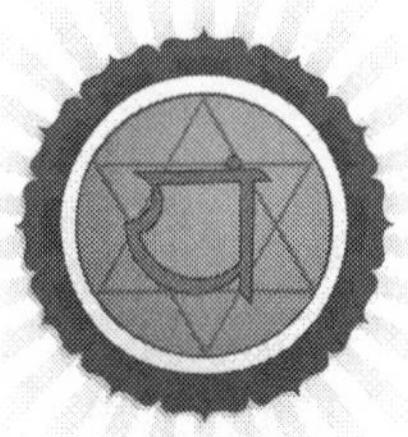

**I LOVE (Anahata)**

The Fourth Chakra rests in line with the heart and emanates the color green. The heart chakra governs the physical aspects of the heart including the thymus, circulatory, respiratory and cardiac systems. It also rules the emotions of love, acceptance and compassion for the self and others, producing an overall sense of oneness with the universe.

- Do I love myself?
- Am I compassionate to those in need?
- How do I express love in my life?

**I SPEAK (Vishudda)**

The Fifth Chakra is on the throat and resonates with the color blue. The throat chakra rules communication, self-expression and creativity. It is associated with the vocal cords, mouth, throat, ears and thyroid gland. When we feel balanced in the throat chakra we feel ease communicating our thoughts.

- Do I share my thoughts with ease?
- Can I stand up in front of a group and give a lecture?
- Can I communicate my creative thoughts to those around me?

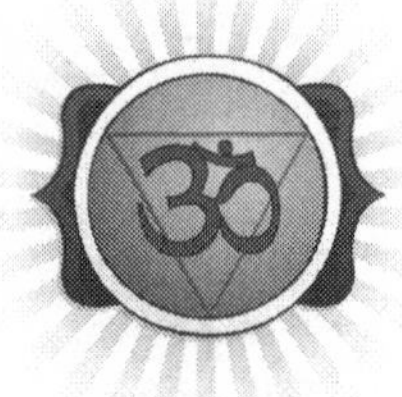

**I SEE (Ajna)**

The Sixth Chakra sits between the eyebrows in the "third eye center" and emanates the color purple. On a spiritual level, the third eye chakra rules our perceptions and intuitions about the world around us, supporting clarity of thought and vision. This chakra is strengthened by meditation. Associated organs include the medulla, pituitary gland and eyes.

- Do I trust my intuition?
- Can I see a clear path to attaining my vision?
- Do I have a strong meditation practice?

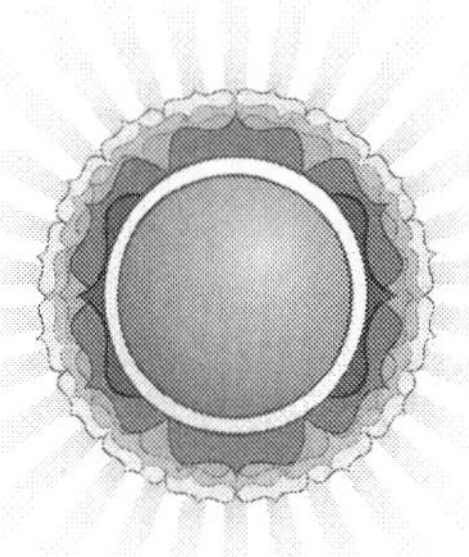

**I UNDERSTAND (Sahasrara)**

The Seventh Chakra or crown chakra is at the top of the head and emanates the color violet. Spiritually, the health of this chakra represents the ability to understand and develop our psychic abilities including intuition. Physically, the crown chakra impacts our pineal gland, cerebral cortex and skull.

- What are my spiritual beliefs?
- Have I experienced déjà vue?
- When I listen to my intuition do I notice it manifesting in my environment?

Along with self-inquiry, energetic medicine can help to release patterns that may be holding us back, contributing to a general lightness of being. In Doris Cohen's book, *Repetition: Past Lives, Life, and Rebirth*, she helps her clients to look at energetic patterns that have been with us for many lifetimes and may be impacting our decisions and actions in the present day. She believes through understanding past life connection, the present day and future can be transformed. In her book and during personal counseling sessions, Cohen provides her clients with rituals to release the past.

Walter Makichen shares a similar philosophy having worked with many clients whose "spirit babies" have shared past lives with one or both of the parents. In sessions with couples, spirit babies have revealed past issues that are preventing them from entering the body from fears of abandonment to the physical threat of animals in the household.

Though not "mainstream" in their approach, both Doris Cohen and Walter Makichen offer insight into vibrational medicine and how--by looking at healing through a different lens--old patterns can be released, resonance restored, and healing can occur.

# Step 5: Align the Spine

When the desire is to enhance reproductive function, be gentle. There is no need to push the body to the edge of exertion, but rather it is important to focus on replenishment. The true place of healing is when we can rest our minds, drop into our experience and let our bodies regenerate. Fully relaxing into the experience is a great challenge for many of us, but experiencing this shift from yang (outward) living to yin (inward) living is where true healing is possible. Too often our minds get in the way of our physical healing by trying to control the process and will something to happen. Sometimes, through movement and bodywork, we are able to release old patterns without having to mentally examine them. By manipulating the positioning of the body and sending fresh blood supply and oxygenation to the organs, the energetic lines of the body are cleared.

Remember, creating new habits requires discipline to entrain your body to follow new patterns. In this case, the discipline is to nourish your body and to choose those activities that allow you to restore and raise your inner vibration. As we discuss various modalities of bodywork and movement, you may notice that you resonate with some styles more than others. Take this opportunity to explore the ones that speak to you until you find your personal groove of self-nurturance.

## Entraining the body to resonate with your fertile vibration

*Begin with the breath.* Many of us run through each day holding our breath in our chests, never once taking a deep inhale or exhale. Our breath is a wonderful tool for bringing us back into the present moment: "A state of Being as opposed to something we do."[xlix] The action of breathing into the belly literally settles our nervous system by impacting the receptors in our gut. Though the concept sounds quite simple, the practice of taking deep breaths must be repeated over time to train the body to release its chest-breathing habit. As Thich Nhat Hanh states in his book, *Happiness: Essential Mindfulness Practices*, conscious breathing is, "the key to uniting body and mind, and bringing the energy of mindfulness into each moment of our life."[l] Conscious breathing is incredibly important, and can be a wonderful tool for challenging situations, such as blood draw appointments, IUI's and transfers. The breath is incredibly powerful, but in order to utilize this skill, you must practice. Harnessing the breath can be practiced at any time during the day. You just need a few quiet moments.

Realize as Thich Nhat Hanh states that, "In the beginning, you may notice that your breathing may feel labored or awkward. Your breath is a result of your body and feelings. If your body has tension or pain, if your feelings are painful, then your breath is affected. Bring your attention to your breath and breathe mindfully."[li] Begin by practicing deep belly breathing when you have free moments during the day or in the morning and evening while in bed. Let the practice be gentle, without forcing the process. Eventually the habit will follow you in your daily life, and you will notice the power of being able to shift instantly out of stress and into calm.

Tip: Thich Nhat Hanh suggests using a simple mantra where you inhale on one word and exhale on another word. Some examples he offers are: [lii]

*In, Out.*
*Deep, Slow.*
*Calm, Ease.*
*Smile, Release.*
*Present Moment, Wonderful Moment.*

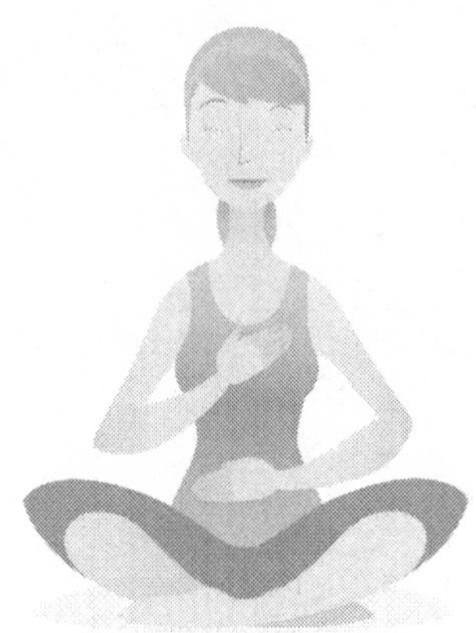

## Movement

Vibrationally moving the body helps to clear energetic pathways and release what is no longer serving, by clearing the mind (releasing emotional toxins) and clearing the body (releasing physical toxins). Physically, exercise invigorates fresh blood and oxygen flow to your reproductive organs, releases feel good endorphins, and optimizes your weight while reducing stress. Ideally, take some time each day to move your body. A simple thirty minutes of exercise each day is enough to feel a shift in vitality.

The most important part of exercise is finding something you love to do. There is a tendency to think of exercise as laborious, and for many the image of forcing oneself to the gym to run on a treadmill and lift weights first comes to mind. However, when exercising for fertility, pleasure is key. In fact, keep in mind that the goal is to replenish the system through expansion rather than draining energy through contraction. Picture the difference between deep belly breathing and weight lifting. The breath expands, while excessive sit-ups contract. The goal is to constantly be in the mode of expansion and supporting our deepest baseline energies. Begin to think of movement as a gift you give yourself each day, by choosing activities that you look forward to.

**Exercises to enjoy and what to avoid for fertility by FertileFoods.com**

Apart from some of the staples like walking, swimming and hiking, here are some favorite fertility exercises you might try:

Qi Gong- a great moving meditation that connects you to the earth, while opening the various energy lines in your body (referred to as meridians in Chinese Medicine)

Product Recommendation:
Tao Yin, The Fertile Soul Qi Gong practice, is designed specifically to improve the communication between the brain, pituitary gland and reproductive organs and reduce stress. Available at http://www.thefertilesoul.com

Dancing- what better way to open your hips and pelvis than with a NIA class? This full body workout is done barefoot and requires no dance technique whatsoever. It is truly a "choose your own adventure" dancing experience.

To find a class near you visit:
http://www.nianow.com

Yoga- fertility yoga helps to calm the nervous system and encourage blood flow to the uterus and ovaries. With increasing popularity, you may be lucky enough to find fertility yoga classes locally.

If you can't find a class nearby, there are several DVD's worth checking out: The Fertile Soul of Yoga, Pulling Down the Moon, Bend, Breathe and Conceive, Yoga 4 Fertility.

Some Activities to Limit:
Excess abdominals and sit-ups- since fertility and getting pregnant is all about expanding your belly, it's best not to over constrict that area. While avoiding over-contracting the abdominals, rest assured that all types of exercise encourage gentle abdominal toning.

Hot yoga- although some women can do hot yoga all the way through pregnancy, you might consider moving to a gentler practice. Heated yoga can dehydrate you and is over-exerting for some. Consider a gentler practice and be sure to drink lots of water.

## Fertility Yoga

Fertility yoga is a highly desirable activity for enhancing your chances of conception. The practice of yoga is known to elicit the relaxation response, an essential element to supporting reproductive function, especially now that the links between stress and infertility are being corroborated by science. What we know is that when stress is perceived physiologically, stress hormones, including cortisol, ACTH, nor epinephrine and epinephrine are released into the bloodstream by the sympathetic nervous system and hypothalamic-pituitary-adrenal axis, forcing the body into "survival mode."[liii] In a state of fight-or-flight, vital functions are prioritized over reproductive function. A constant surge of stress hormones over time interferes with hormonal balance and ovulation patterns.

What is interesting is that "the same influences that the organism is most likely to interpret as emotionally stressful are, not surprisingly, also the most powerful psychic triggers for the HPA axis: psychological factors such as uncertainty, conflict, lack of control, and lack of imagination are considered most stressful stimuli and strongly activate the HPA axis. Sense of control and consummatory behavior result in immediate suppression of HPA activity."[liv]

What this research indicates is that though there may be many elements in our lives that feel out of our control, it is essential to have practices in your life that feel within your control to counteract the fight-or-flight reflex and reduce stress. Another study by Harvard researcher Alice Domar PhD showed that 55% of infertility patients who participated in her mind-body program for a 10-week period (which included yoga and meditation) conceived, compared to 20% in the control group when tested after one year.[lv] Mind-body techniques such as yoga have also been shown to improve in vitro fertilization success rates by lowering stress hormones.

Beyond reducing stress, fertility yoga helps to support conception in the following ways:

- Increases blood flow to the reproductive organs
- Opens the pelvic and hip region
- Aligns the spine
- Releases toxins
- Releases emotional tension
- Regulates the endocrine system
- Elevates mood
- Relieves insomnia

## The Fertile Secret's daily fertility yoga flow

### Intention Setting

Sitting cross-legged, place your hands in prayer position at your heart center, eyes gently closed. Breathe deeply into your belly and take a few moments to set an intention for your practice. What would you like to draw to yourself today?

Note: Make sure you are comfortable. Feel free to use a blanket under your sacrum or sit on your knees if that feels better.

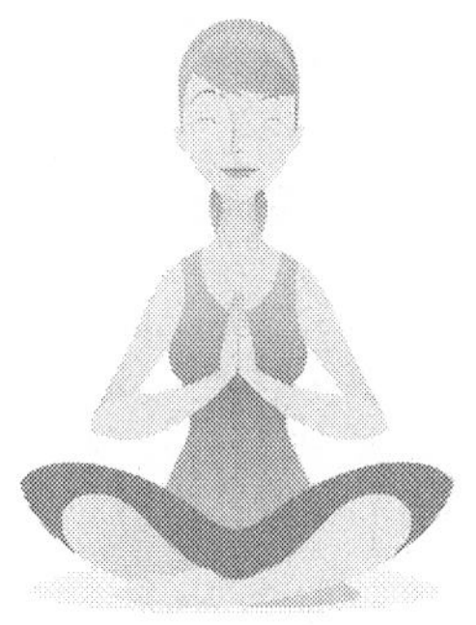

### Fertility Breath

Keeping your eyes closed, place one hand on your heart and one hand on your belly. On the inhale, feel the chest expanding. On the exhale, allow the belly to fill. Repeat this breath slowly at least 10 times.

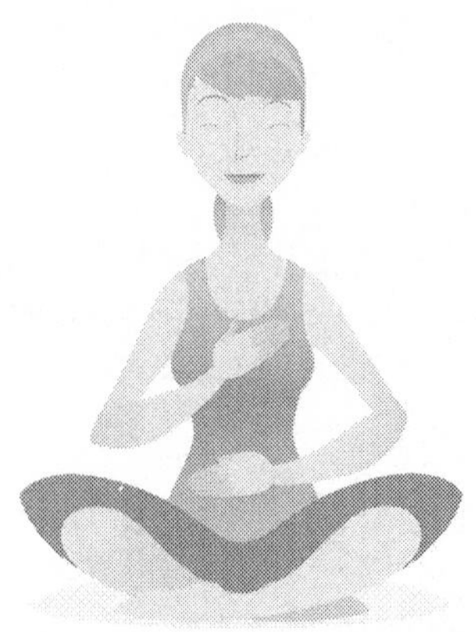

**Body Circles** (right, then left)

Let your eyes open and place your palms facedown onto your knees. Begin to move in circular motions to the right, releasing the body completely. Once you have completed five full circles, move to the left and do the same.

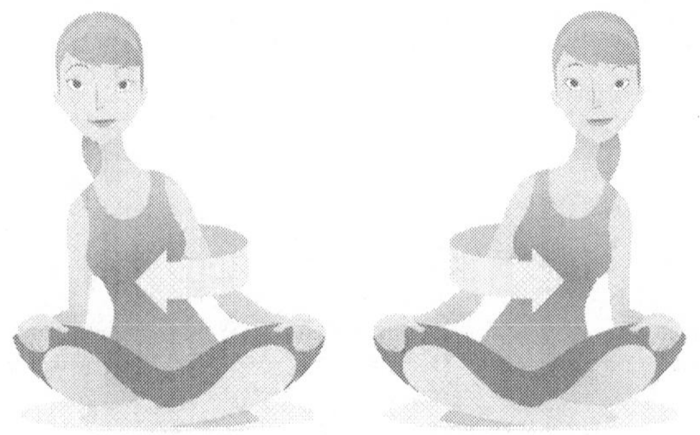

**Arch Forward, Retreat Inward** (forward and back)

Once you have completed your circular motions, spend some time expanding and contracting the heart center. First, press against the knees as you expand the chest forward, feeling the stretch across the front of the body. Next, drop your head and arch the back, allowing the heart to drop in. Repeat this movement, slowly waking up the spine, at least 5-10 times.

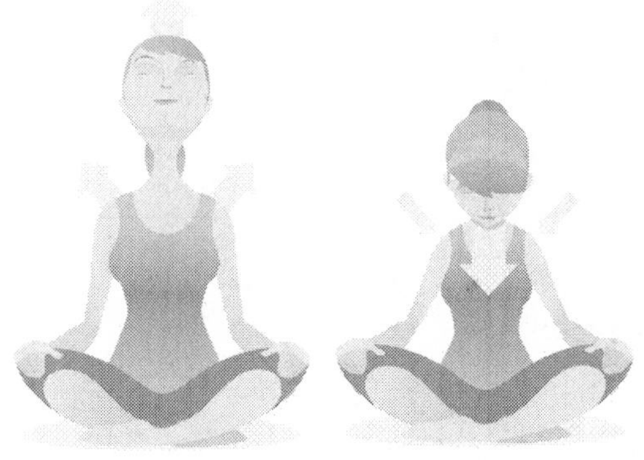

**Cat Cow Stretch**

Come onto your hands and knees, with palms flat on the floor, arms directly underneath your shoulders and knees hip-width apart. Inhale, and press into your palms. Lift up through the belly and arch your back like a cat. On the exhale, press into the palms. Lift your eyes to the sunlight. Arch the back, and draw the chest forward. Repeat this motion 5-10 times using the breath as your guide.

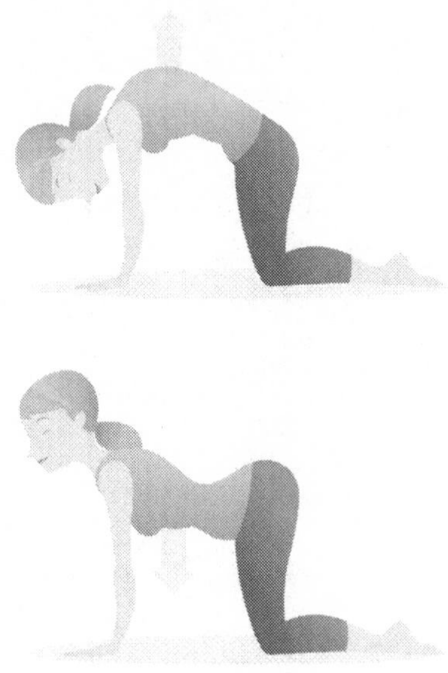

**Gentle Rolling on the Back**

Roll onto your back, and pull your knees to the chest. Allow yourself to rock from side to side, forward and back and in small circular motions. The sacrum area has many beneficial acupressure points that support fertility.

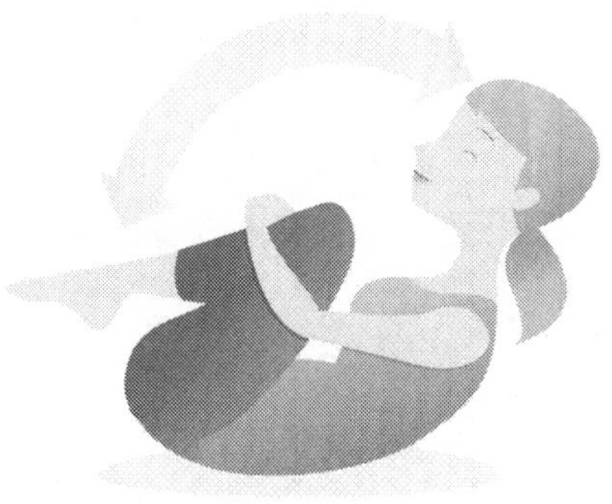

**Wind Removing Posture**

Reach your left leg out in front of you, back of the leg on the floor. Draw your right knee in towards the armpit, using your exhale breath to drop in a little deeper each time. After 5 slow breaths, repeat your right side.

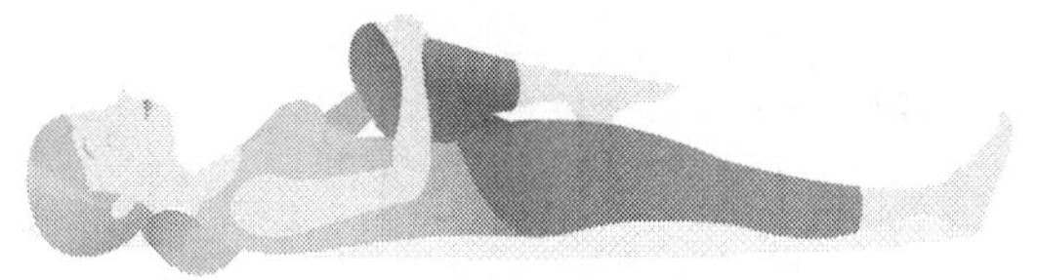

**Twist** (except during your luteal phase)

Draw your right knee in towards your chest. Place the left hand on the outside of the right knee and let the weight of the leg drop you over to the left side. Let your right arm extend and gaze over the right shoulder if it is comfortable. Use your breath to drop in a little deeper, and feel the deep stretch across your chest, hips and in your spine. Repeat on your left side.

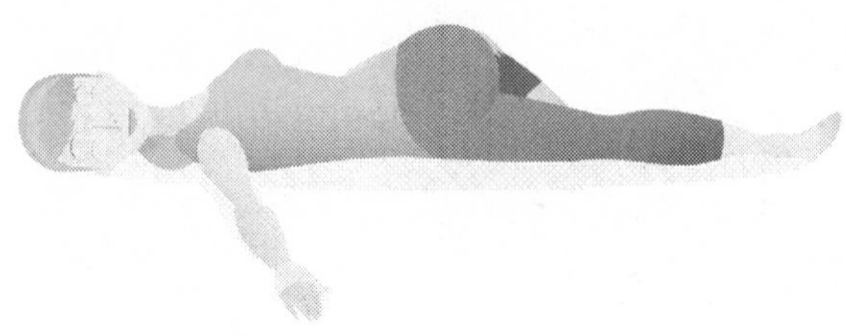

**Legs Up on the Wall** (except during menses)

Moving into deep relaxation, find a wall and sit with your right shoulder and hip touching the wall. Begin to lie down on your back, while simultaneously lifting your legs up onto the wall, and scooting your buttocks towards the wall. Let your arms drop to the side, palms facing up, open to receive. Breathe gently, and give yourself a few minutes to drop into this posture before moving to final savasana.

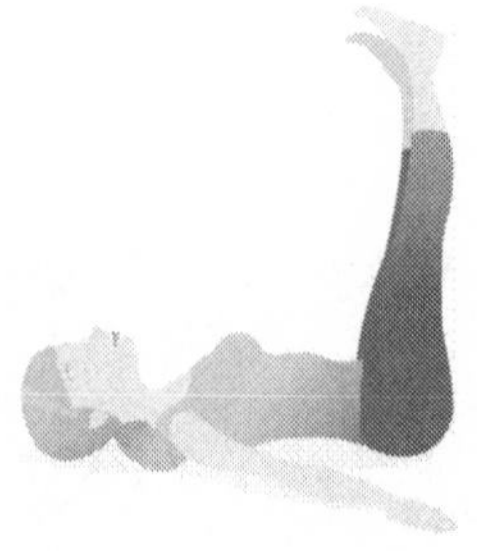

**Savasana**

For final relaxation, lie on your back with palms facing up. You may want to place a bolster (or a couple of blankets) under your knees to increase comfort and cover yourself if you are feeling cool. There is nothing to do here but drop in and relax. Give yourself 5-10 minutes here; this deeply relaxing posture is the most important.

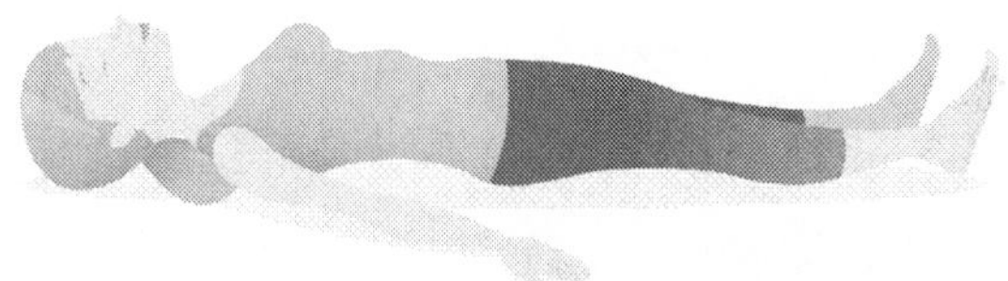

## Bodywork

Treatment Options:

**Chiropractic**
Since the nerves that correspond with fertility run through the spine, it makes sense that identifying any "subluxations," or spinal distortions, could improve reproductive function. Research on the topic is currently under way, and early indications look promising.[lvi]

**Craniosacral Therapy**
In craniosacral therapy, the practitioner uses gentle

touch to manipulate the skull and sacrum bones. The technique aims to reduce blockages on all levels: physical, emotional, mental, and spiritual, to reduce stress and clear energetic pathways in the pelvic region. Craniosacral is particularly helpful in supporting fallopian tube mobility and health.[lvii]

**Reflexology**

Reflexology treatments target specific points on the hands and feet that are linked to the major organs of the body. Practitioners believe that through the massage, energetic pathways are cleared in the body to enhance fertility. One study showed that pregnancy rates increased with reflexology treatment as did menstrual cycle and ovulation patterns.[lviii] A new study, currently in the works, will compare the benefits of reflexology to the ovulatory drug chlomiphene in a study of 150 women over a three-month period.[lix]

Human touch is powerful beyond measure. The Touch Research Institute [TRI] in Miami has reported numerous healing occurrences connected to the power of touch: "Studies have shown massage to have a positive affect on conditions from colic to hyperactivity to diabetes to migraines, in fact, every malady TRI [Touch Research Institute; in Miami Florida] has studied so far.[lx] Physical touch encourages the body to release oxytocin, contributing to increased pleasure. We live in a society where touch is often feared. As a result of our "touch phobic" society, some of us are deprived of the human connection and power of healing touch that could be experienced through something as simple as a hug. In my offices, I have developed a daily ritual called "the huggle." During this practice our office comes together as a group to receive energy, encouragement and connection. It is a show of human kindness that has had a positive impact on our daily operations.

Besides making a point of reaching out and connecting physically with those who are close to you, getting regular bodywork is essential on the healing journey. It has been long understood that massage has the power to reduce stress. In a study published in the International Journal of Neurosciences (2004), researchers studied the effect of moderate, light or vibratory massage on stress levels by studying brain waves and heartbeat. All three groups reported decreased stress and anxiety, the largest drop being in the moderate pressure group. Since fertility massage is only indicated in the first half of the cycle (the follicular phase), relaxation massage is often used in the second half of the cycle (the luteal phase) to alleviate common physical and emotional constraints that women experience during that time frame. Sometimes, when a client is primarily dealing with the stress of infertility, they may experience more benefit from a relaxation massage rather than focused belly work. The meditative practice of massage works on both a physical and emotional level to invigorate blood flow and release feelings of fear, increasing receptivity to the implantation process. At my wellness center, CNY Healing Arts, aromatherapy is often used alongside massage to maximize relaxation, while detoxifying lymph, supporting circulation, reducing anxiety, regulating stress hormones and releasing any stored trauma.

## Massage for fertility

(Adapted from *Rainforest Home Remedies: The Maya Way to Heal Your Body and Replenish Your Soul*, by Rosita Arvigo and Nadine Epstein)

"At the very heart of Maya medicine is the concept that medicine is all around us. We pass it daily right on our very doorstep; we also find it at roadsides and in trees, plants, stones, animals, dreams, and prayers. The Earth Mother is the great wellspring of medicinal power."lxi
— Rosita Arvigo

Rosita Arvigo is the founder of the Arvigo Techniques of Maya Abdominal Massage (ATMAM). In her book, *Rainforest Home Remedies: The Maya Way To Heal Your Body and Replenish Your Soul*, Rosita speaks of the traditions she learned from Don Elijio Panti, a traditional Maya Shaman, and describes the practice of maya abdominal massage as a "medical religious" healing modality steeped in the rich traditions of the Maya people.[lxii] ATMAM is based on two principles:

1. **Homeostasis**, which is the body's innate ability to self-regulate, heal, and regenerate.
2. **Hemodynamics**, involving "the flow of arterial and venous blood, nerve impulses, lymph and Qi."

Many cultures are intrigued by the blood flow and the life force energy contained within it, which the Mayas have named Ch'ulel. It is within the Ch'ulel that the soul-- comprised of 13 parts--resides, and it is known that an imbalance in any one of the 13 parts of the soul must be restored for true healing to occur.[lxiii] Life force is primarily diagnosed by pulse assessment that offers a clear picture of a patient's physical and spiritual condition.[lxiv] Maya pulse diagnosis is very similar to Chinese medicine with the addition that the Maya traditions repeat prayers for healing while taking the pulse at the wrist, feeling for eighteen different variations of beat, depth and intensity.

## What can you expect from your first Maya Abdominal Massage treatment?

For women, your practitioner will customize your bodywork according to the stage of your menstrual cycle, using deeper lower belly work during the follicular phase (before ovulation), and focusing on relaxation during the luteal phase (after ovulation). It is important to avoid direct lower belly massage after ovulation on months when you are trying to conceive. When you receive a positive pregnancy test, you will want to wait until the second trimester to resume ATMAM. In women, the pelvic region and reproductive organs tend to hold a lot of emotions. You can expect your massage to be cleansing and detoxifying, physically and emotionally, leaving you with a deep sense of mental peace.

**Maya Abdominal Massage benefits fertility in the following ways**

- Increases blood flow to the reproductive organs
- Nourishes follicles with fresh blood supply and oxygen
- Helps to break down scar tissue and adhesions
- Helps to resolve blockages in the fallopian tubes
- Re-aligns the uterus, as in the case of a prolapsed uterus
- Relieves stress and anxiety, releasing emotional blockages
- Improves digestion and absorption of nutrients
- Reduces inflammation due to PCOS, endometriosis, cysts or fibroids
- Addresses cramps and heavy bleeding
- Regulates enlarged prostate
- Improves sperm quality and quantity: sperm count, motility and morphology

- Aids in a prolonged labor or preterm labor
- Restores healthy menstrual flow in amenorrhea
- Improves, tones and cleanses uterine lining
- Helps to prepare body to carry a healthy pregnancy, a key ingredient in the case of frequent miscarriages

**When to receive Maya Abdominal Massage**

*Men and Women:*

For best results, start ATMAM 90 days before beginning ART, and commit to a minimum of one treatment per month from ATMAM practitioner in conjunction with a self-care routine at home. Men can receive ATMAM anytime, but women have special considerations depending on the time of the cycle, ART treatments and contraceptives.

*Special instructions for women:*

Receive ATMAM after your period and before ovulation, trigger shot or retrieval. If you are in the process of doing a donor cycle, you can have a Maya Abdominal Massage anytime before transfer. In the case where you are taking birth control pills due to cysts, you can receive ATMAM anytime, which may help to resolve your cysts very quickly.

Maya Abdominal Massage uses a holistic approach that considers four aspects in the healing process, including uterine position, herbal medicine, spirituality and emotional states.

## Uterine Position

"The uterus is the woman's center. If her uterus is not in proper position and good health, nothing in her life will be right. She will be as out of balance as her uterus." [lxv]
— Don Elijio Panti

Maya Abdominal Massage uses healing abdominal work to reposition the pelvic organs and treat a pro-lapsed or tilted uterus. Massaging the abdominal region can also help to break up any adhesions or blockages that may be preventing conception. It is estimated that adhesions are a contributing factor in nearly 40% of infertility cases.[lxvi] If you have had injuries such as falls or accidents to the hips or sacrum, traumas such as surgery, sexual abuse or difficult childbirth or car accidents, your body reacts to the experience and holds the trauma until it is released. These memories become muscular tensions, and structural changes that all impact the position of a woman's uterus. When the uterus or any of your organs are out of alignment, the entire system is impacted: blood, circulation, lymph flow, the nervous system which helps to communicate hormones, your energy flow, and distribution of vital nutrients and energy.

As CNY Healing Art's certified massage therapist, Erin McCollough, reminds us:

*"Just like we clean our house, our bodies need constant maintenance as well. ATMAM gives people the tools to maintain and provide optimal reproductive health. Infertility allows us to take an introspective look at our bodies and do an internal house cleaning. ATMAM is a time-honored tradition for physically, emotionally and energetically revitalizing a man or woman's body."*

A woman's uterus can take on a number of different positions, which can often be realigned by ATMAM. In Mothering magazine, Catherine S. Gregory explains how the various uterine positions can impact a woman's menstrual cycle and ultimately her fertility.[lxvii]

A side-lying uterus often corresponds with ovarian function, often leading to ovarian cysts, hormonal imbalance, challenges with conception and irregular or no ovulation (annovulation).

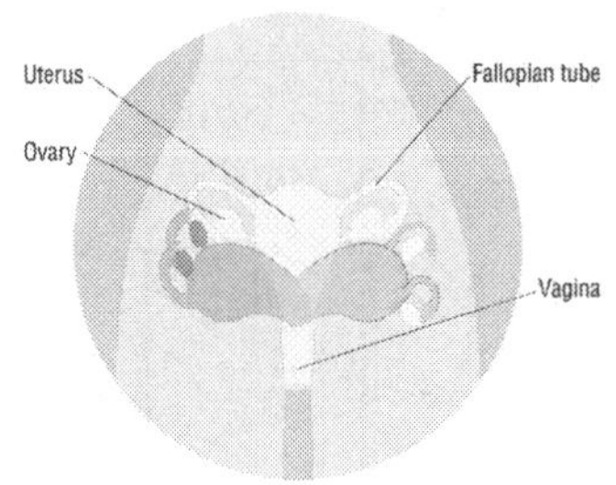

An anteverted (forward lying) uterus may be a culprit in bladder infections, frequent urination and urinary tract infections.

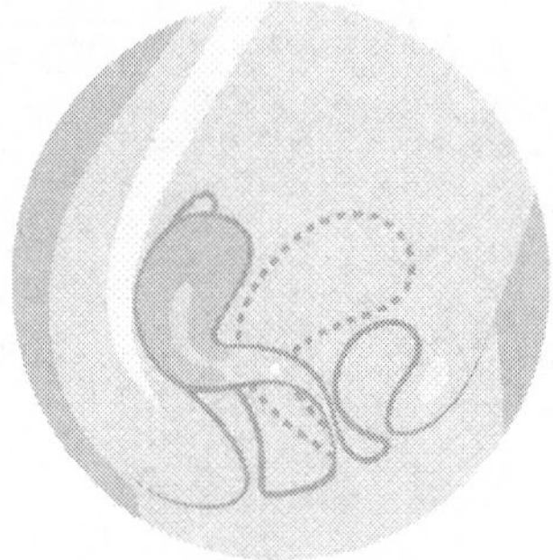

Dotted line indicates properly positioned uterus

A prolapsed (low-lying) uterus may be implicated with issues with bowel and bladder incontinence, painful intercourse and varicose veins.

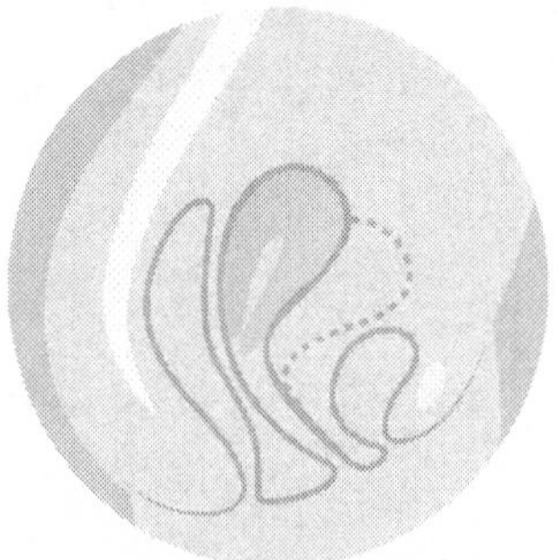

Dotted line indicates properly positioned uterus

A retroverted (tipped back) uterus may put constraint on the bowel, leading to constipation and can also put pressure on the sacral nerves leading to low back cramping and increased cramping during menses.

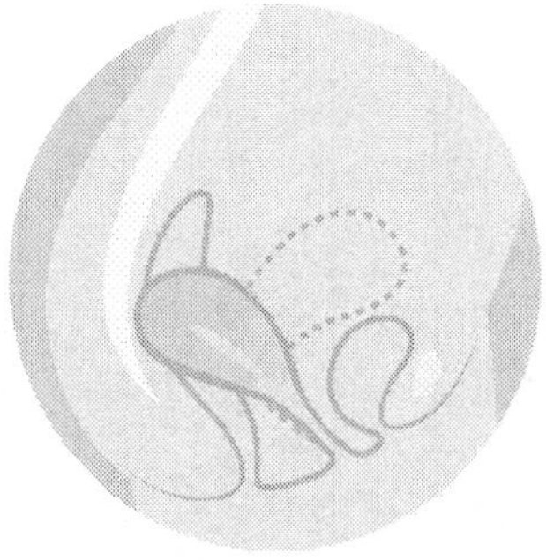

Dotted line indicates properly positioned uterus

## Causes of Uterine Misalignment

- Carrying heavy loads just before or during menstruation or too soon after childbirth
- Running on cement surfaces
- High heel shoes
- Sacral injury from fall, car accident or other
- Poor pelvic alignment
- Constipation
- Carrying a child on the hip for prolonged periods of time
- Emotional trauma such as rape, abuse or incest
- Aging and the natural pull of gravity

- Walking barefoot
- A career in dancing, aerobics or high impact sports
- Frequency of pregnancy in close proximity

The Arvigo Techniques address clients with a holistic approach to health and wellness considering four aspects in the healing process, including uterine position, herbal medicine, spirituality and emotional condition. Practitioners of these techniques are from a variety of professional backgrounds, providing this modality within their scope of practice.

**Herbal Medicine**

"Medicinal plants can be prepared as teas, made into tinctures in alcohol, steeped in oil to produce a healing salve for the skin, dried and powdered for wounds, boiled with sugar to make syrups, mashed with salt to make poultices, and administered as herbal baths. Medicinal plants can also be dried, powdered, and rolled into cornhusks and smoked." [lxviii]

The Maya believe that every plant carries within it an innate intelligence. Herbal medicine carries with it deep beliefs such as the ceremonial planting of a grain believed to bring abundance.[lxix] The process of collecting and preparing the herbs involves a prayer that acknowledges the great gift of each plant. Through a combination of prayer and intention, these plants become allies and work with us to bring healing and balance.

**An ancient Maya prayer**

In the name of God the mother, God the father and God the Holy Spirit, I am the one who walks in the mountains collecting plants to heal the people. I give thanks to the spirit of this plant, and I have faith with all my heart in its great power to heal.

In general, plants and foods are divided into hot and cold formulas created to bring equilibrium back to the body's temperature, which governs the health of the individual. Contextually, "cold ailments exhibit chills, cramping, paralysis, or constipation. Hot ailments exhibit fever, diarrhea, vomiting, boils and red skin rashes."[lxx] Some of the most common herbs used in Maya medicine include:

"Hot" plants and herbs: amaranth, oregano, orange leaves, chocolate and onions.
"Cold" plants and herbs: dairy, nopal, limes, lemon grass, and purslane.

**Spiritual: Spirits and Prayers**

"I am the one who collects and prepares the medicine, but it is faith that cures." [lxxi]

Beyond the physical experience of the massage and the plants, it is faith and prayer that guide the principle of this medicine. The spirits of Maya medicine are believed to work alongside practitioners and are activated by prayer. As the hands are on the body or simply collecting the herbs, prayer is held for healing of the body. This intention, as we know, magnifies healing impacting the experience and outcome of both patient and practitioner.

**A prayer for spirits to assist in the healing process:**

In the name of God the mother, God the father and God the Holy Spirit. I pray to God and the Maya Spirits with my prayer to heal______________. I ask God to help her and I ask a favor of the Maya Spirits that they would help her also. I have faith with all my heart in the great healing power of this prayer, the plants, the baths.

## Emotional: Mind-Body Connection

Simply by being present, a practitioner serves as a guide to assist in the creation of an environment where the client can truly let go. When clients feel safe to express themselves they can release negativity that may be building up in their physical and emotional bodies and draining their system of vital life force. Intuitively listening to the client, lending compassion to them and offering "commonsense advice" plays an enormous role in releasing what no longer serves their greatest health and good.[lxxii]

## The Arvigo Techniques of Maya Abdominal Therapy™: "Self Care Massage"

Although it's best to work with a trained Arvigo practitioner, anyone can learn the self-massage technique described here. You may experience some temporary changes in menstruation, including a heavier blood flow or an increase in the number of days of flow. This is a sign that your uterus is cleansing. If you become pregnant, stop self-massage and seek the advice of a trained Arvigo practitioner for prenatal massage techniques.

To locate an Arvigo workshop and/or practitioner in your area, go to *http://arvigotherapy.com*.

## CAUTIONS and CONTRAINDICATIONS:

While this technique is safe when applied appropriately, there are times when direct massage over the uterus is contraindicated. **Do not perform direct massage on your uterus if you: are pregnant**, have had abdominal surgery within the last six months, are under medical treatment for cancer or pelvic infection, or wear an intrauterine device (IUD) for birth control. Do not continue with self care massage if you should experience pain or emotional upheavals during the treatment, are taking any painkillers that might mask pain during treatment, or experience a sudden onset of pain. Refer to your health care provider or Arvigo Practitioner for appropriate evaluation.

**SELF Care Massage**

- Wear loose, comfortable clothes. Empty your bladder. Lie on your back, with support under your knees.
- Relax and breathe deeply for several minutes.
- Bring both hands together on to the pubic bone. Tuck one thumb under the other, with the other eight fingers close together. Fingers should be slightly bent and relaxed so that your hands resemble a hoe.
- Slide your hands off the pubic bone toward your naval, and sink your fingers as deep into the soft flesh as is comfortable.
- On your next exhalation, firmly stroke in an upward motion halfway to your navel. Remember to breathe slowly and exhale with each massage stroke. Repeat this upward movement of your hands, from pubic bone toward navel, for about two minutes.

- If you experience discomfort, reduce the pressure but continue to massage upward and within your comfort zone. If you experience any tenderness after the massage, give yourself a few days' rest before resuming self-massage, using a lighter touch.

**- The Arvigo Institute, LLC**

**Week 13: Maya Abdominal Massage by CNY Fertility client and blogger April All Year**

When many of us think of a massage, we think of relaxation and escape. The Maya Abdominal Massage, though it does provide relaxation, is not necessarily an escape and works to re-balance the spiritual center (uterus). According to the article, "A Time-Honored Alternative: Maya Abdominal Massage," by Jill DeDominicis, MAM helps treat infertility and other issues, (irregular menstrual cycles, ovarian cysts, digestion, headaches, etc.), by, "addressing and removing blockages in the abdominal area for better chi flow throughout the body." MAM also works to correctly position the uterus to ensure there is more blood flow to the area and enhances circulation to the ovaries and fallopian tubes. If any of you have been told you have a tipped uterus, MAM also addresses this issue, which may indirectly impair fertility.

Additionally, MAM flushes toxins from the body, aids in digestion and helps restore hormonal balance. (See http://arvigotherapy.com for additional information.)

To date, I have received two complete Maya Abdominal Massages and one partial treatment, because I had a urinary tract infection. (Yes, I was told that perhaps I was a bit too active before ovulation – sometimes we just can't win, ladies!) Since the actual massage is a deep tissue treatment, which works on the abdominal organs, there was a possibility the infection would spread. However, I was able to undergo the meditation part of the treatment, which requires a bit of emotional work on the patient's end.

From a patient perspective, there are three segments of the MAM treatment. First, the patient lies on her stomach while the therapist massages the back and upper neck and then adjusts the legs and back in a way that reminds me of chiropractic care, but is gentler. Next, the therapist will have you lay on your back so s/he can complete the deep tissue abdominal massage. This includes a series of repeated exercises that work to properly position your uterus and clear any blockages. Obviously, adjusting a uterus' position is no easy task and requires a skilled MAM professional. Thus, patients must only seek treatment from properly qualified practitioners, especially since part of the therapist's goal is to teach you to perform

MAM self-care independently. Self-care requires patient work and commitment. It is recommended that patients perform MAM on themselves from the date their menses stops up to the date of ovulation. Personally, this self-care treatment only takes twenty minutes, which is not a considerable chunk of time; yet, I have not been as dedicated as I should be, but that is a topic for another week.

Finally, the meditation segment of the treatment takes place, and your therapist will leave you to listen to a guided meditation for approximately 30 minutes. The guided meditation plays on the stereo, and encourages you to focus on what is requested of you for the half hour. Regardless of the specific meditation, the guided exercise fosters spiritual growth by providing a safe and productive outlet to address personal issues that may be interfering with various aspects of your life. While most of us would prefer to pretend as though our emotional baggage is non-existent, the guided meditations do offer an opportunity to let go of fear and negativity and also serve as a way to communicate with one's inner self. Also, during the meditation segment, your therapist may treat you with castor oil by placing a cloth soaked in castor oil on your stomach and then placing heat on top of the cloth.

Remember that MAM is about becoming physically healthy and spiritually intact. Both men and women benefit from MAM and should remember to seek out qualified professionals. Overall, it is important to commit to a series of MAM treatments, (a minimum of three is recommended,) and to perform the self-care exercises. Since MAM has been proven to increase fertility along with improving overall health, you may want to consider giving this option a try.

Blessings,
*April All Year*

# Step 6: Balance with Traditional Chinese Medicine

A message from Dr. Randine Lewis, Ph.D., L.Ac., founder of The Fertile Soul:[lxxiii]

"Coming from a Western background and education, it was initially difficult for me to accept the theories of traditional Chinese medicine (TCM). I was asked to change the way I thought about life, the human body, the entire universe. I found myself arguing with my TCM professors until one of them told me to forget all the ideas of Western medicine that I had come to accept as the only truth. What a challenge—to put aside my scientific background and allow for new ideas and a different paradigm! It was odd to shift my thought process from scientific, linear thinking to a more associative way of thinking—especially when we were talking about medicine. If I hadn't seen these techniques work for me personally, I would have walked out. The attitudes of Eastern medicine toward health, disease and the world seemed too strange, almost like a unique religion.

While it didn't make sense, what I was learning was fascinating. After all, I thought, TCM has worked for millions of Asians for thousands of years. And it helped me get pregnant naturally when my Western doctor's only solution was to use drugs like Clomid. I decided I was ready to learn everything about traditional Chinese medicine that I could, especially as it related to infertility. So I applied myself, learned how to use the principles of Chinese medicine with patients, and watched their astonishment as they too became pregnant when Western medicine had given them no hope.

Now I am grateful for both my Western and Eastern training, because it allows me to serve not only as a healer, but also as a bridge between the two medical worldviews. I understand and value the ability of Western medicine to quantify every moment of a woman's reproductive cycle, to pinpoint exactly where the potential lack of harmony might be. I also value enormously the technological wizardry of Western science, the technology that allows us to see inside the body with great accuracy, to use microsurgery to repair the smallest tears and blockages, and above all, to use assisted reproductive techniques to allow women with no hope of conceiving to bear children.

At the same time, I also see the wisdom and benefit in cultivating our body's innate healing abilities, and of nourishing ourselves--body, mind and spirit--to preserve and extend our health. Eastern medicine is empowering; it recognizes the role each of us plays in shaping our health, rather than seeing it as being up to a trained professional to "fix" us. In my experience, the miracles that are possible when we harness our healing power are almost without limit."

— Dr. Randine Lewis

## Chinese philosophy

Traditional Chinese medicine has been used for thousands of years to treat imbalances in the body and prevent disease. In ancient times, the village doctor made his living by keeping the villagers healthy and the only time he was not paid was when one of his patients became sick. Eastern medicine is one of the earliest forms of preventative healthcare that values keeping the patient well through balancing the energy of the body. When the body becomes out of balance, diseases like infertility can occur.

"Tao is not an answer to the question, "What should I do?" but a response to the question, "How do I do it?" This knowing how — how to heal, how to grow, how to live, how to rediscover my self and my origin — is an ongoing process, a way to walk through our lives rather than a static thing or way to be. It is a stone rolling down a hill, a leaf falling from a tree, light replacing shadow as the sun rises above the tops of the trees. Tao makes a space in the known where the unknown can happen. Poised right here, right now, at the place where I stand, Tao is the ongoing ever-imminent, ever-astonishing arising of the possible." [lxxiv]
— Lorie Dechar

## The concept of Qi

According to TCM, Qi (Chi) is the life force energy from which everything formed and formless is created. The concept of Qi is cross-culturally known as "shakti" or "prana" in India, "ka" in Egypt, "ki" in Japan and "mana" in Africa. The fundamental principle of Chinese medicine is that free flowing Qi is the determinant of vital health, and any stagnancy in the energy flow will lead to imbalance and disease. A Chinese practitioner's primary purpose is to re-establish this free flowing Qi and remove stagnancies through use of acupuncture, acupressure, herbal medicine, and Qi Gong and Fung shui.

There are many kinds of Qi that exist within us and are also available to us in our natural surroundings. When we are born we come into the world with Yuan Qi (ancestral Qi), and throughout our lives we gather nourishment from food, air, water and energetic practices that endow us with Hou tain qi (post-natal Qi). We are each composed of the fundamental sources of masculine energy (Yang-Qi,) and feminine energy (Yin-Qi). Wei-Qi (protective Qi) covers the surface of the body, protecting our immunity. Qi flow is measured by its ability to flow through the meridians of the body, some of the most common being Spleen Qi, Kidney Qi, Liver Qi, Heart Qi and Lung Qi.

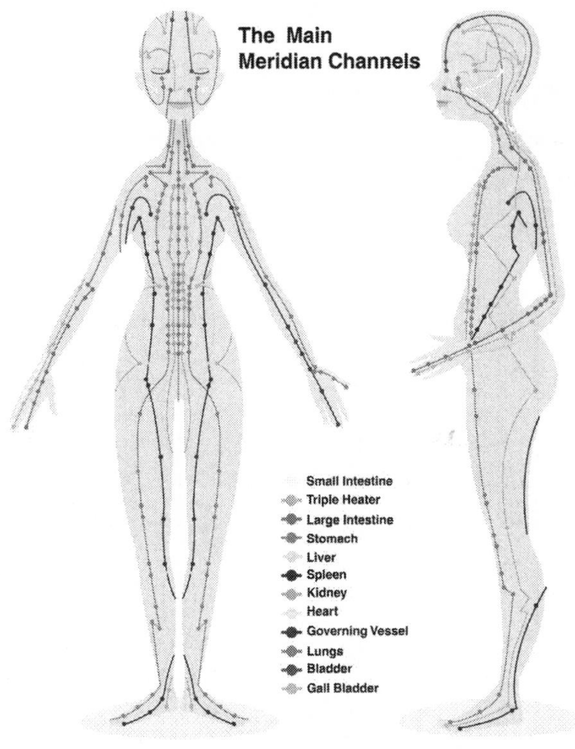
The Main
Meridian Channels
Small Intestine
Triple Heater
Large Intestine
Stomach
Liver
Spleen
Kidney
Heart
Governing Vessel
Lungs
Bladder
Gall Bladder

## Yin, yang and your body

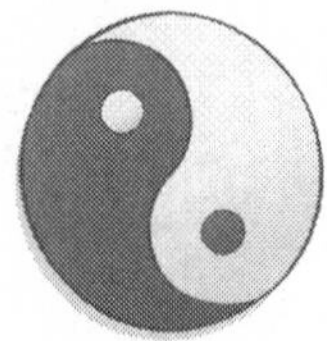

The image of the yin and yang symbol is probably one of the most popular modern symbols of balance, and we are indeed a culture in need of balance. With the invention of Internet, e-mail, instant messaging, Facebook and Twitter, we have become creatures of instant gratification, where 9-5 is a distant memory and the expectation of instantaneous answers has become the norm. We are outward (yang) focused beings and are being asked to go inward (yin) to find our balance.

We are constantly being influenced by how we relate to yin and yang. When these opposing forces are in balance, we feel healthy, and when they are out of balance, we are more likely to experience illness.

To understand yin and yang, we look to the opposites we see in our environments and how the balance of those polarities creates synthesis in our lives.

| Yin | Yang |
|---|---|
| Dark | Light |
| Moon | Sun |
| Water | Fire |
| Passive | Active |
| Descending | Ascending |
| Female | Male |
| Contracting | Expanding |
| Cold | Hot |
| Winter | Summer |
| Interior | Exterior |
| Heavy | Light |
| Bone | Skin |
| Front | Back |
| Interior of body | Exterior of body |

Yin and yang are likened to a candle, where yin is the wax and yang is the flame. The wax nourished the flame's ability to burn brightly, but once it is gone, the light is extinguished. Like the candle, we are born endowed with all the essence or "congenital Jing" we have to carry us through our lives and fuel our activities. In a balanced lifestyle, women are believed to have an excess of energy to support a growing child, but our habits and the nature of our environment tends to deplete our reserves.

**Activities that deplete our essence and fertility include**

- Lack of sleep
- Over exercise
- Excessive work
- Lack of nutrients
- Too much stress
- Toxins
- Alcohol
- Prescription drugs
- Caffeine

Simply put, fertility is a receptive yin state, and our habit of putting too much energy into our external world can drain our inner energies. According to the principles of TCM, we can replenish our inherent fertility by adjusting our lifestyles to include more yin activities that promote restfulness and diminish stress. The simple act of repeating the yin-yang self-inquiry exercise from Chapter 1 helps us to stay in integrity with our energy input and output, reminding us to devote more energy inward.

## The five elements of your fertility

TCM practitioners use a five-element theory to understand the pathology and physiology of the human body in relationship with our natural environment. By looking to the elements of nature in relationship to each of our organ systems, Chinese medicine aims to restore balance by viewing each element as an important part of the greater whole, where symbiotic relationships are essential for balanced health.

The Nourishing or Shen cycle (clockwise circle) depicts how nature and our bodies work in unison to create balance. In the symbiotic relationship of the nourishing cycle, each element is considered the mother of the next: **water** nourishes the **wood** to grow, **wood** fuels our **fires** to burn, **fire** creates ashes to become **earth**, **earth** yields **metal**, and **metal** is heated creating vapor and condensation, which becomes **water**.

The Regulating or Ko Cycle (clockwise pentagon) illustrates the cycle of imbalance that is perpetuated when elements take over control in nature and our bodies. The destructive cycle shows **water** extinguishes **fire**, the heat of **fire** melts **metal**, **metal** cuts through **wood**, **wood** contains **earth** and **earth** absorbs **water**.

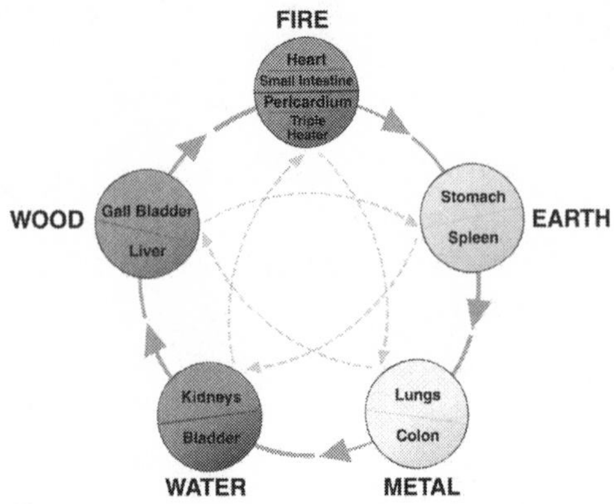


The five elements are used as a diagnostic tool to observe patterns in the body or propensities in the individual towards specific imbalances based on his or her constitution. Constitution is determined by looking at various correspondences of each element, including as they relate to the individual and the environment: season, climate, yin and yang organ systems, sense, tissue, emotion, personality characteristics and taste. A diagnostic pattern may in part be derived from a practitioner's observation in any and all of these areas. For example: a female client who appears very angry, with a green tint to her skin, sharp pain under her right rib cage, complaining of PMS in the spring would clearly be experiencing an imbalance in her wood element where the liver channel would be treated and balance restored. Though we may be dominant in one or several elements, we each consist of all five elements. To optimize or restore our fertility, we must aim to create balance in body, mind and spirit.

| Abbreviated Table of Correspondences | | | | | |
|---|---|---|---|---|---|
| | WATER | WOOD | FIRE | EARTH | METAL |
| Season | Winter | Spring | Summer | Late Summer | Autumn |
| Climatic Qi | Cold | Wind | Heat | Damp | Dryness |
| Yang Organ | Bladder | Gallbladder | Sm. Intestine | Stomach | Lg. Intestine |
| Yin Organ | Kidney | Liver | Heart | Spleen | Lung |
| Sense Organ | Ears | Eyes | Tongue | Mouth | Nose |
| Body Tissue | Bone | Sinews | Blood Vessel | Muscles | Skin |
| Emotion | Fear | Anger | Joy/Shock | Worry | Sadness |
| Color | Black | Green | Red | Yellow | White |
| Taste | Salty | Sour | Bitter | Sweet | Spicy |

**The Fire Element Meridians:** Heart (yin), Small intestine (yang), Pericardium (yin), Triple warmer (yang)

The fire element represents the heart and is considered the emperor of the entire organ system. Every other organ is meant to serve the heart, so it can sit on its throne and focus on circulating blood through all the vessels.  A person with a dominant fire personality is charismatic: the social center of every party.  Constantly on the go, quickly moving from event to event, a fire personality risks "burn-out" which can result in anxiety, insomnia, restlessness and lackluster in the eyes. Fire personality types thrive when they incorporate cooling environments with an abundance of relaxing activities to counteract the constant buzz. General health complaints related to the fire element include palpitations, hypertension, heart problems, sores on the mouth and tongue. The most common fertility related disorder associated with the heart is Premature Ovarian Failure (POF) viewed as a lack of communication between the heart and the uterus.

**The Wood Element Meridians:** Liver (yin), Gallbladder (yang)

The wood element represents the liver and the gallbladder pairing, viewed as the general who directs initiatives and action, having the 360-degree perspective to make educated decisions. A person with a dominant wood personality is a pioneering decision maker, plowing through obstacles to bring vision and results. Unafraid of standing up for what they believe in, wood personalities will not back down from arguments or uncomfortable confrontation. The level of stress in their lives often brings about a level of constraint that manifests itself as Liver Qi stagnation. This is characterized by a constriction in the blood flow that stops the liver from properly processing hormones, resulting in PMS, irritability, excessive frustration, headaches, bloating, irregular cycles, fibroids, heavy bleeding, digestive issues and hormonal imbalance. Conversely, in a person that lacks wood energies can be indecisive, without direction and the ability to properly express emotions, resulting in liver blood deficiency associated with a lack of blood flow as in amenorrhea, abdominal pain, masses in the abdomen, irregular menstruation, painful menses and dark clots in menses.

**The Metal Element Meridians:** Lung (yin), Large intestine (yang)

The metal element includes the lung and the large intestine pairing. Those who have dominant metal personalities are conscientious, self-disciplined and organized. These personalities thrive in a structured environment where they feel a sense of "control" over the environments. The metal energies are about holding on and letting go as with the breath (the lung), and discharging waste (the large intestine). When lung energies are deficient, a person may feel overly critical, grief stricken, overwhelming sadness and unable to let go. Lung deficiency may present in conditions including asthma, allergies, frequent colds and constipations. Since the skin is the corresponding tissue, rashes, sweating disorders and eczema are also related to lung deficiency. Issues of control reflect autoimmune conditions related to fertility including recurrent miscarriage.

**The Earth Element Meridians:** Spleen (yin), Pancreas (yang)

The earth element includes the spleen and pancreas, governing digestion, blood production and immunity. Those with dominant earth personalities are grounded, nurturing, compassionate and quintessential mediators. These personalities thrive in environments where they can "mother" and are recognized for their love of bringing people together and feeding them. The earth energies are about boundaries and the balance of conserving energy and sending it outward. When earth energies are imbalanced, earth personalities may become meddlers, over-worry with a feeling of heaviness, clouded thinking and often finding it difficult to get rid of excess weight. In Spleen Qi deficiency there is an inability to absorb and properly distribute nutrients to all the other organs in the body often partially caused by food sensitivities and resulting in overly heavy menses or light menses, a lack of energy, muscle tone, IBS, gas, bloating, food sensitivities, canker sores, and heartburn. Dampness or accumulation of phlegm is also common, characterized by cysts, as in the case of PCOS. Evidence is now showing that malabsorption conditions like celiac disease may be an underlying cause in infertility.[lxxv]

**The Water Element Meridians:** Kidney (yin), Bladder (yang)

The water element includes the kidney and the bladder, corresponding elements of the adrenals and the reproductive organs, responsible for circulating our store of baseline energies of yin and yang. A water personality is the ultimate philosopher, one who appreciates the depths in quietude and research and would prefer to spend time alone. In balance, these personalities are fearless, determined and powerful in the pursuit of their goals. They thrive in environments that promote trust and are diminished by fear and paranoia. The water energies contain our very essence and are most impacted by stress or the perception of stress and lack of safety and security. Kidney imbalances are most associated with ovulation difficulties along with lower back pain, water metabolism, fertility and sexuality. A person may appear fearful, or withdrawn with dark circles under their eyes. Kidney yin in particular declines with age and the process is sped along by elements of heat or stress in our lives resulting in hot flashes, cessation of menses, night sweats, and dry skin. Kidney yang is compromised when there is a lack of warmth generated in the body resulting in frequent urination, cold extremities (which signals a lack of blood flow to the uterus and ovaries), low libido and incontinence.

## Treatment with Chinese medicine

### Acupuncture

Acupuncture is an ancient Chinese healing practice that has been used for thousands of years to prevent illness and treat imbalances in the body. Acupuncturists insert tiny, sterile needles into specific acupressure points to improve the flow of energy and remove any blockages creating disease. *The Fertile Secret* acupuncture program uses the healing benefits of Traditional Chinese Medicine on its own or combined with assisted reproductive medicine to restore balance in your body and help to reverse infertility. *The Fertile Secret* acupuncture program can be used alongside fertility treatments and ideally to improve egg quality during the three months prior to conception.

**What can I expect in my first acupuncture treatment?**

During your first visit, your fertility acupuncture specialist will assess your areas of imbalance and create a specialized program using a combination of acupuncture, herbal remedies and lifestyle recommendations. Your first treatment will last approximately one hour and will include a full intake and acupuncture experience. If this is your first time receiving acupuncture, you may be surprised to learn that acupuncture is painless and deeply relaxing. Many people begin to notice the physical and emotional benefits of acupuncture after their very first session: from improved sleep patterns to reduced pain and increased energy.

**How does acupuncture help fertility?**

Acupuncture and Oriental medicine benefit fertility in the following ways: [lxxvi]

1. Regulate menstrual cycle
2. Improve sperm count and motility
3. Reduce stress and anxiety associated with infertility
4. Normalize hormone and endocrine systems
5. Improve blood flow in the uterus
6. Decrease chance of miscarriage
7. Increase the chance of pregnancy for women undergoing in vitro fertilization (IVF)

**Research**

A recent study in the British Medical Journal revealed that women doing in vitro fertilization treatments were 65 percent more likely to conceive when they used acupuncture in conjunction with their western medical treatment.[lxxvii] Additional studies support the significance of acupuncture for the outcome of assisted reproductive medicine.[lxxviii]

- Acupuncture administered on the day of embryo transfer significantly improves the reproductive outcome of IVF/ICSI.[lxxix]
- Acupuncture is associated with higher clinical pregnancy rates and live birth rates.[lxxx]

**Acupressure for fertility**

The principles of acupuncture can be applied from

the comfort of your own home, using the healing energy present within your hands. Using the pads of your fingertips, experiment with putting light pressure on each point for 30 seconds to start. Notice some points will feel especially good, and you may feel drawn to linger longer. Using acupressure helps us to become more in tune with the source of energy we can tap into at any moment. The following are general points to use to enhance your fertility through therapeutic touch at home.[lxxxi]

## Reproductive Acupressure Points[lxxxii]

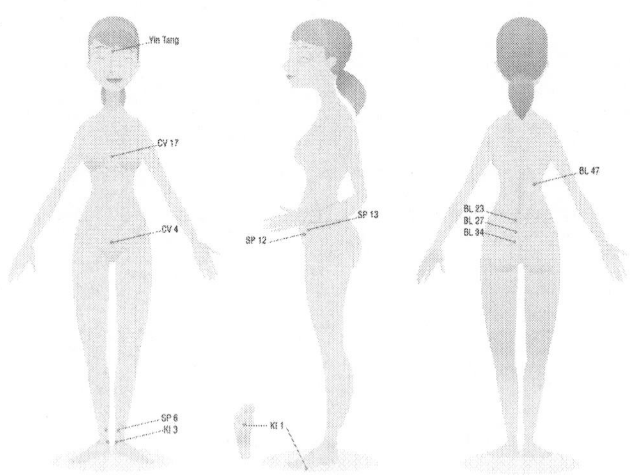

| Location | Name | How to Locate | Benefits |
|---|---|---|---|
| SP 12 & 13 | Rushing Mansion/ Mansion Cottage | Pelvic area between crease in leg and trunk of the body | Relieves impotency, menstrual cramps, abdominal discomfort |
| B 23 & 47 *do not use with degenerative disks | Sea of Vitality | 2-4 finger widths from the spine at waist level in line with the belly button | Relieves pelvic constriction, reproductive problems, premature ejaculation, fatigue backaches |
| B 27 - 34 | Sacral Points | Perimeter of sacrum | Relieves sterility, urine retention, sacral pain, sciatica, impotency |
| CV 4 | Gate of Origin | 4 finger widths below the belly button | Relieves impotency, uro-reproductive problems, irregular menstruation & discharge |
| CV 17 | Sea of Tranquility | 3 fingers above breastbone | Balances emotions, calms spirit, relieves nervousness, depression & grief |
|  | Yin Tang | Point between eyebrows | Relieves depression, irritability, confusion, stimulates |

| | | | |
|---|---|---|---|
| | | | immune system & calms spirit |
| K 1 | Bubbling Spring | Base of the ball of the foot between the two pads | Stimulates kidneys, reproductive organs and rejuvenates spirit |
| K 3 | Great Ravine | The depression midway between the anklebone and Achilles tendon | Restores the reproductive system |
| SP 6 | Three Yin Crossing | 4 finger widths above the anklebone, behind the bone | Regulates menstruation and treats reproductive disorders |
| REN 4 | Gate of Origin | 4 finger widths below the belly button | Supports conception by building energy |

# Step 7:
# Nourish Your Cells

(Adapted from *Cooking for Fertility: Foods to Nourish Your Fertile Soul* and FertileFoods.com, by Kathryn Flynn)

We each have within us trillions of cells that are constantly looking for optimal nutrients to keep our bodies vital and alive. Every hour million of our cells divide, and when they do, they utilize stored energy in our bodies in the form of vitamins, minerals and antioxidants from the food we eat and our supplements. When the nutrients are not present, the cells borrow or steal from another healthy cell, leading to oxidation and degeneration. Chronic degenerative diseases, like infertility, are more prevalent now than ever in part, perhaps, because many of us are simply not well nourished. Whether it's due to the degradation of our soils, over-consumption of packaged and processed foods, environmental toxins, or simply a lack of fresh air and sunlight compounded by stress, it is most important to find simple ways to nourish us each and every day.

Along with a strong foundation in daily relaxation and movement, food is the fuel we use to fill up our tanks and give us energy to go about our daily lives. The types of foods we use can drastically impact our energy, our state of mind and our health. In fact, food has been used as medicine for thousands of years to treat and heal disease and illness. Since it's something we partake in on daily basis, it actually has more power to create health than many of us believe. Simple changes the food choices we make can improve reproductive function. Learning to make healthy choices without sacrificing taste and pleasure is the key to improving energy levels, digestion, hormonal balance and optimizing your weight. By taking a holistic approach to your dietary practices, you create the foundation for living a fertile life.

## #1: Find your healthy weight

We know for sure that finding your healthy weight can go along way to supporting balanced hormones and healthy reproductive function. According to the American Society for Reproductive Medicine (ASRM), twelve percent of all infertility cases are a result of either weighing too much or too little. The BMI (body mass index) is a wonderful tool for calculating where you are in terms of your weight: underweight, normal, overweight or obese. Though there are many factors, including one's build and muscle mass, that can impact the relevance of the BMI index, it is generally a good ballpark indicator of where you are with your weight now and helps you to gauge how to achieve your healthiest weight. To calculate your BMI:[lxxxiii]

**Imperial BMI Formula**

$$\text{BMI} \, (kg/m^2) = \frac{(\text{weight in pounds} * 703)}{\text{height in inches}^2}$$

| BMI | Weight Status |
|---|---|
| Below 18.5 | Underweight |
| 18.5 - 24.9 | Normal |
| 25 - 29.9 | Overweight |
| 30.0 & Above | Obese |

Dietary changes also have special significance in helping to treat PCOS. Studies have shown that weight loss, through diet and exercise, as little as 5-10% can be helpful in restoring fertility. A low-calorie diet can help balance the menstrual cycle, re-instate ovulation and reduce prevalence of male hormones. When obesity is a factor in PCOS, 30% of women have been reported to experience amenorrhea. In women of normal weight only 4.7% did not have a monthly cycle.[lxxxiv] Being underweight can be equally problematic, as eating disorders have been shown to rob the body of vital nutrients and fat stores so necessary to hormone production. What is most important is to adopt a healthy, balanced lifestyle by being moderate with your eating and exercising.

## #2: Balance your blood sugar levels[lxxxv]

One of the best things you can do for your health is learn to balance your blood sugars through lifestyle and dietary choices. When blood sugar levels are balanced, all else starts to fall into place: your energy levels soar, hormones balance out, your mood stabilizes and extra weight drops off effortlessly.

Blood sugar levels get out of control quickly when we exist on a diet that consists mostly of simple carbohydrates and sugar. Consider the consequences of a typical breakfast: a bagel and orange juice. Physiologically our blood sugar spikes, notifying our body to release insulin. Insulin's job is to bring our blood sugar back down. Oftentimes, our blood sugar goes too low, requiring our body to release cortisol, a stress hormone, to bring it back up to normal. When this pattern repeats itself continually, we develop what's called "insulin resistance." Our body is tired, and insulin regulation no longer works well. Physiological feelings include: hormonal imbalance, low energy, and inability to lose weight, "puffiness" and depression. If we do not heed the body's warnings, insulin resistance may progress to "metabolic syndrome" where our symptoms become measurable by Western medicine. Risks include a higher waist circumference, heart disease, high cholesterol and blood pressure, among others.

Ideally, we want to reverse this entire process before it gets out of hand and leads to diabetes. Here are some steps you can take to increase your insulin sensitivity and manage your blood sugar levels:

1. Cut out simple and refined carbohydrates like white bread, flour, pasta and packaged, processed foods. Choose whole grains, fruits and vegetables as the staples of your diet.
2. Avoid excessive sugar from candy, soda, concentrated fruit juices. Use agave nectar and xylitol as low glycemic alternatives.
3. Eat protein, carbohydrate-balanced meals, and snacks regularly throughout the day.
4. Choose low glycemic foods with an index of 50 or less (white bread = 100).
5. To help you make the change, consider Usana's high fiber, low glycemic RESET cleanse to detoxify your body, break your sugar cravings, reset your insulin sensitivity and recalibrate your metabolism.

## #3: Stay hydrated with water, herbal teas and by avoiding coffee[lxxxvi]

Our bodies are made up of 97% water. We could go without food for x days but without water we would die within x days. The rule of thumb is to drink at least half of your body weight in ounces of room temperature (easier to digest) water per day and avoid dehydrating substances like coffee. Replacing coffee with herbal teas is important for several reasons. Most recently, Kaiser Permanente released findings of a 2008 study that determined the equivalent amount of caffeine in two cups of coffee increases your chance for miscarriage. Caffeinated beverages include coffee, hot chocolate and energy drinks. Dr. De-Kun Li, the study's lead author, confirms that, "caffeine is dangerous during pregnancy, because it can cross through the placenta to the fetus and it can be difficult for the fetus to metabolize the caffeine. Caffeine may influence cell development and decrease blood flow to the placenta."[lxxxvii] Beyond threat of miscarriage, both caffeinated and decaffeinated coffee contain volatile oils that tax the liver. Since our livers are primarily responsible for metabolizing reproductive hormones, it is important to keep them working optimally. Tea, on the other hand, has many healing benefits and can be used to support sleep and relaxation (chamomile), digestion (peppermint and ginger), fertility (red raspberry), and to help gently detoxify the liver (lemon and milk thistle).

## #4: Eat an Asian-based diet and favor warming foods over raw foods[lxxxviii]

Modeling an Asian diet may just be one of the best ways to balance health and nutrition. The Chinese eat 30% more grains than Americans do and have significantly better health rates, including lower incidence of breast cancer and heart disease. Rather than treating meat as the main dish, the Asian style of cooking treats meat as a condiment; where your plate is mostly filled with steamed vegetables, some grains and a palm sized portion of protein with some healthy fats (think olive oil or avocado). Moderation is key.

Beyond what you are eating, the digestive system must also be respected to allow proper absorption and distribution of nutrients to all the organs. Imagine for a moment that your digestive system is a cooking pot stoked by a fire. To keep the fire, the temperature must remain relatively high and be protected from adverse conditions like rain and dampness. Your internal fire functions in much the same way, where everything you put in your mouth will either support or impede your digestion. Consider the impact of cold ice water or ice cream on your digestion. As soon as it hits your digestive system, the fire is quelled, impacting your body's ability to absorb nutrients and distribute fuel for organ function. If you have eaten a large meal, a sludge may form, slowing the digestive process and potentially leading to constipation and indigestion.

Ideally, we want food to transform quickly into usable energy, which enables the reproductive system to function optimally. For this reason, choosing cooked foods is preferable to raw foods. Raw foods are best consumed in the warmer months or for shorter periods of detoxification. Though gentle detoxification can be helpful to fertility, our first priority is to build a strong foundation through deep nourishment. When you want to enjoy salads, chew your food well and slowly to activate digestive enzymes.

## #5: Choose organic, fresh, colorful foods over processed and packaged

There is an innate wisdom to choosing organic local foods closest to the source. Reflect for a moment on the difference between an orange that has sat on a shelf for days, versus picking a fresh orange from a tree. The vitality in the latter can be seen in the vibrancy of the orange and taste in its juice. Beyond supporting your local community, eating in sync with what nature gives us automatically connects us to the seasons and natural flow of life. Dehydrated, packaged foods with preservatives are unnatural to our bodies and add unnecessary chemicals to our systems. Non-organic products have been treated with pesticides and hormones that our foreign to our bodies ecosystems and have the potential to wreak havoc on our hormonal system, leading to conditions of estrogen dominance, including but not limited to endometriosis, polycystic ovaries and fibroids.

The solution is to choose organic products whenever possible and consume a diet of natural foods: vegetables, fruits, grains and hormone-free vegetable and animal proteins. Visit your local organic grocer or weekly farmers market each week or more frequently if you can. Choose a colorful array of foods, this way you will ensure that you are getting all of the nutrients you need. Load up on cruciferous vegetables (such as broccoli and cauliflower) containing di- indolymethane (DIM), a compound that stimulates more efficient use of estrogen by increasing the liver's ability to metabolize excess estradiol. When you can't find organic produce, soak your fruits and vegetables in 2 teaspoons salt, ¼ cup of vinegar and a quart of cold water for 10 minutes to remove unwanted pesticides and critters.

## #6: Avoid artificial sweeteners and the sugar rollercoaster[lxxxix]

Most of us would agree that at one stage of our lives or another, a sweet treat was the "staple" that got us through the day. Coffee and chocolate are the "pick me ups" of choice for so many of the women I work with. The scenario goes something like this: quick energy pick-up, push through current activity and crash. It's the typical sugar rollercoaster that feels energizing in the moment, and ultimately leads to burnout if relied upon for long periods of time.

Deciding to quit sugar and artificial sweeteners is one of the best choices we can make for our health. Over-consumption of refined sweeteners can lead to blood sugar imbalances, mood swings and malabsorption of vitamins including minerals and calcium essential for fertility. It's actually quite natural to crave sweets when we are feeling down because they do replenish our bodies with a momentary blast of serotonin. Unfortunately, it's not a sustainable dose, and when the pattern is repeated over time, our brains keep telling us we need more of our substance of choice to continue feeling good. Eventually we can't get enough to bring the natural high and we must look to healthier options to boost our serotonin.

Quitting the sugar fix can seem daunting at first, and it is most important to not overly restrict, which can lead to feelings of deprivation and binges. However, a period of detoxification is likely necessary before moving on to moderation. A great program for kicking the sugar cravings, recommended by Dr. Christiane Northrup in her book, *Women's Bodies, Women's Wisdom*, is Usana's 5 day RESET cleanse. The low glycemic foods and high fiber content help to curb the cravings and set the stage for healthier eating.

Additional tips to cut the sugar cravings include:

- Use natural sugar sources, such as fruit and lower-glycemic choices to help keep blood sugar levels stable and avoid fluctuating hormone and energy levels.
- Eat fruits in their whole form, not as juice. Sweetened juices are loaded with sugar, producing dampness and encouraging yeast formation in the body, and even unsweetened juices lack the fiber that helps slow absorption of natural sugar from whole fruits.
- Avoid foods sweetened with sugar, corn syrup, or artificial sweeteners. Commercially prepared baked goods, pastries and sodas are generally full of white flour, sugars, or chemicals that disrupt your body's natural processes.

**Natural sweetener substitutes:**

Replace 1 cup of refined sugar with:
¾ cup agave nectar
1 cup brown rice syrup
½ cup blackstrap molasses

¾ cup raw honey
¾ cup maple syrup
1 cup Xylitol

- Soft drinks- many sodas contain chemicals like aspartame and high fructose corn syrups. Best to cut the artificial stuff out before, during, and after pregnancy and quench your thirst with water. If you need something a little more exciting, try sparkling juice with a splash of fruit juice.
- Chlorella has a high protein content that can help to curb sugar proteins while fueling your body with the deep nourishment of chlorophyll that helps to manage blood sugar levels.

## #7: Choose sprouted whole grains and consider gluten free[xc]

If you are experiencing any of the following symptoms: bloating, gas, constipation, irritability, depression, fatigue, arthritis, psoriasis, hormonal imbalance or eczema, you may be suffering from a simple food sensitivity. Though often considered a healthy whole grain, wheat is actually one of the eight most common allergens. One of the best ways to discover if wheat is an issue for you is to remove it from your diet for one month and see how you feel. Many people have noticed significant improvements in their health and well being after removing wheat from their diet.

It is important to note that having wheat sensitivity is different than being diagnosed with gluten intolerance. Celiac disease is a chronic intestinal malabsorption disorder caused by intolerance to gluten. It is suspected that 1 out of 111 North Americans could be diagnosed with celiac disease, 20% of North Americans are believed to have non-celiac gluten sensitivity.[xci] Old tests were unreliable; whereas new tests have greater sensitivities showing as much as 1 in 3 have the gene that predisposes them to gluten intolerance.

If you have been diagnosed with gluten intolerance or Celiac's disease, please also avoid the products marked (G). When shopping, it is safe to purchase products marked gluten-free as you are assured they will not contain wheat.

Amaranth, Barley (G), Buckwheat, Flaxseed , Kamut* (G), Millet, Quinoa, Brown Rice, Spelt (G), Sprouted Wheat, Teff Flours, Almond, Tapioca, Chestnut, Chickpea, Hazelnut, Jerusalem artichoke, Sorghum, Oat (G: Gluten-free varieties available), Rye (G), Pastas

## #8: Choose healthy sources of full fat dairy[xcii]

A recent study released by Harvard Medical School, "The Nurses Health Study," shows that women who consume low-fat dairy are more likely to have difficulty conceiving than women who consume whole fat dairy.[xciii] Healthy sources of fat are essential for the building blocks of hormones that are stored in fat cells.

Since a lot of people have sensitivities to the complex protein structure of cow dairy, it is beneficial to look for alternative sources. The effects of cow dairy allergies and sensitivities range from person to person. In a full-fledged dairy allergy, lactose and casein create an adverse response in the immune system, creating a range of symptoms from skin rashes, flatulence and fatigue. Those who are not "allergic" to cow dairy, may still be "dairy intolerant," lacking in the digestive enzyme necessary to breakdown lactose. If you suspect a dairy allergy, consider getting allergy testing or consider cutting dairy out of your diet for four weeks and see how you feel when you add it back in.

Though many of us grew up believing milk was the only way to meet our calcium needs, this is simply not true. Calcium is abundant in many non-dairy, vegan sources including sesame seeds, spinach, collard greens, turnip greens, mozzarella cheese, blackstrap molasses and mustard greens. If you find yourself sensitive to cow dairy, try some of the following milk alternatives:

**Goat milk-** the protein structure of goat milk is less complex than cow dairy and may be easier for your body to digest. The taste is slightly "tangy" and may take some getting used to.

**Hemp milk-** made from the chia seed, hemp milk has the full benefits of omega 3 fatty acids. Hemp milk is a great substitute for morning smoothies and cereals.

**Almond milk-** with a nice nutty flavor, almonds are complete with Vitamin E and offer a great source of protein. Almond cheese offers an interesting twist on the traditional grilled cheese sandwich.

**Soy milk-** is a very popular beverage and a good alternative in moderation. Some research shows that it can interfere with our body's natural estrogen receptors, and therefore it is best to avoid in refined forms like isolated protein powders.

## #9: Cut out toxins including alcohol, nicotine, chemicals in foods, unnecessary medications and street drugs

Knowing that our livers process our hormones and all that we put in our body, it makes good sense to keep our diets simple and clean. Unnecessary toxins in the form of alcohol, drugs and chemicals in our foods force our bodies to work harder than necessary to detoxify. They also deplete our baseline stores of energy better used for reproductive function and overall vitality.

The purpose of eating for fertility is to build up the body. As they say, it takes a lot more work to build a house than it does to burn it down with a single match. When we make the conscious choice to stop ingesting toxins, there is a period of detoxification, where cravings may increase.

During this time, it is important to apply strategies of deep relaxation and self-care to bridge to your most healthy state. The following gentle detoxification tips will help to cleanse the liver, helping the body to process hormones with greater ease.

- As a rule of thumb, choose foods with the least amount of ingredients possible. If you can't pronounce or don't recognize an ingredient, don't buy it.

- Each morning upon rising, drink a hot cup of water with lemon.
- Consume an abundance of dark leafy green vegetables to supply fresh chlorophyll.
- Eat cruciferous vegetables and make use of DIM to rid the body of excess estradiol.
- Sip on yogi detox tea or milk thistle tea.
- Take warm baths with Epsom salts and lavender.
- Consume mostly vegetarian sources of protein.
- Take wheat grass each day.
- Use the following spices when cooking: basil, caraway, cardamom, cayenne, chive, clove, coriander, dill seed, garlic, marjoram, mustard leaf, orange peel, peppermint, rosemary, spearmint, star anise, tangerine peel, thyme, turmeric.

**Fertility Friendly Fast Food Alternatives[xciv]**
**FertileFoods.com**

Don't think you can pass up a big mac combo? I've heard that before, and the only way out of your quandary is to find some equally delicious recipes to satisfy your cravings. Fast food is a habit, and while I'm all about meals to-go, there are certainly some choices that are better than others. If you're craving a quick fix on the road, consider some healthier choices like Panera Bread (great soup and salad), Real Food Daily (for my vegetarian friends in LA), Fresh Direct (a favorite for my NY clients who tell me "recipe" is a bad word), or the Whole Foods hot food bar (my personal favorite). The rest of you might like to try some of these delicious recipes and recreate your burger combo at home.

**Instead of french fries, try yam fries:**
Yams are a lower glycemic variety of potato that not only tastes delicious, but also may be the secret ingredient for pre-conception twin creation. The Harvard Medical School Nurses Study noted that that the trans fats found in a small serving of commercial French fries are enough to adversely affect fertility.

2 medium yams, cut into 1/8 -inch strips
2 tablespoons olive oil
½ teaspoon parsley
¼ teaspoon sage
¼ teaspoon thyme
½ teaspoon rosemary
Sea salt or dulse flakes to taste

Preheat oven to 400 degrees. Slice sweet potato into circles or thin strips. Baste with olive oil, and add spices. Place a single layer on baking sheet, and cook for 45 minutes or until tender inside and crisp outside.

**Black bean burgers:**

Black beans are considered a reproductive tonic in Chinese Medicine and are loaded with protein, fiber, folate, iron and antioxidants all essential vitamins and minerals for your fertility. The Harvard Medical School Nurses study found iron rich foods like lentils to support ovulation and fertility in women.

1 cup black beans
1 small carrot, chopped or grated
1/3 cup onion
¾ to 1 cup crushed gluten-free crackers
2 to 3 cloves chopped garlic
1 tablespoon herb de Provence
Sea salt to taste
1 tablespoon black sesame seeds
2 to 3 tablespoons unrefined olive oil

Place all ingredients in food processor and pulse until thoroughly combined. Form mixture into patties or smaller "cakes." If they are not holding together because they are too "wet," add more crackers. Place in an oiled skillet and cook 5 to 7 minutes on each side or until browned. Serve with Ezekiel sprouted grain buns.

**Opt for natural sodas:**
Instead of drinking soda, substitute the following combination of juice and sparkling water to offer a fizzy satisfaction. By doing so, you will avoid harmful chemicals that disrupt the proper release

and regulation of hormones, and benefit from the natural nourishment of fruits and water.

½ cup limeade, lemonade or any unsweetened juice
½ cup sparkling water

Combine ingredients in a tall glass and enjoy! Store bought varieties to try: Reeds Gingerale (made with real ginger), Izze sparkling juice (delicious flavors), closest to cola: Zevia

## #10: Supplement with antioxidants and supplementation

Stress, pollution, chemical exposure and over-medication all cause free radicals to form in our bodies, which deplete our cells of essential nutrients necessary to keep us healthy and free of chronic degenerative disease, including infertility. It's a simple equation: the more free radicals your body produces, the more antioxidants you need.

In fact, supplementation is most important to support reproductive function and a healthy pregnancy. Deficiencies caused by the typical American diet, dense in highly processed foods, may contribute to sub-fertile states particularly deficiencies in vitamins A, C, E, B complex, zinc, and selenium.

To ensure you are getting all that you need, eat a nutrient-rich diet and supplement with quality vitamins. Please note that all vitamins are not created equally and it is worthwhile to investigate the rating of your prenatal vitamin in the Comparative Guide to Supplements, a research study commissioned by the Canadian Government to help consumers choose quality supplements.

**Supplementing with food and vitamins for fertility**

Choose a **prenatal vitamin** that contains 1000 mcg of folic acid along with your basic antioxidant support:

**Vitamin A** or beta-carotene- carrots, butternut, sweet potato, broccoli, spinach and apricots

**Vitamin E-** olive oil, almonds, sunflower seeds, olives, papaya, blueberries, peanut, spinach, kiwi, broccoli, mango, collard greens and avocado

**Vitamin C-** citrus fruit, berries, papaya, red bell peppers, broccoli, strawberry, cantaloupe, kiwi, cabbage, spinach and sweet peppers

**Zinc-** wheat germ, lean meat, pumpkin seeds and seafood

**Selenium-** Brazil nuts, wheat germ, molasses,

sunflower seeds and eggs

**Vitamin B12 food sources-** fermented soy products, seaweeds, alga, salmon, shrimp, halibut, beef, lamb and liver

**Folate-** fortified breakfast cereals, legumes, lentils, chickpeas, collard greens, papaya, peas, asparagus, broccoli, strawberries, oranges

**Additional basic supplements:**

**Fish oil-** for neural function and development

**Omega 3 food sources-** Usana optomega oil, menhaden, salmon, cod liver, cod, shrimp, tuna, pink salmon, king crab, mackerel, flax, flaxseed, hemp, hemp nuts, canola, walnuts and pumpkin seeds.

**Calcium for bone density**
Calcium food sources- hijiki, wakame, kelp, kombu, wheat grass, sardines, agar agar, nori, almonds, amaranth, hazelnuts, parsley, turnip greens, brazil nuts, sunflower seeds, watercresss, garbanzo beans, quinoa, black beans, pistachios, pinto beans, kale, spirulina, collard greens, sesame seeds, Chinese cabbage, tofu, walnuts, okra, salmon, eggs, brown rice, milk products, bluefish, halibut, chicken, ground beef, mackerel

**Iron for anemia**

Iron food sources- alfalfa, arame, broccoli, cherries, garbanzo bean, kale, micro-algae, parsley, seaweed

## #11: Eat with pleasure and mindfulness[xcv]

Often times when men and women confront changing their diets, there is a feeling of impending doom and restriction that greets them. Culturally, this is associated with the very word "diet," which implies going without our favorite foods and having to sacrifice. The principles of eating for fertility are altogether different. Since fertility is about expansion, the most important step in making dietary changes is to practice pleasure and mindfulness as you explore various alternative food choices. What you are likely to discover is that after a short while is that your taste buds will change and your cravings will adjust. Along the way, allow yourself to indulge in cravings from time to time, following the 80/20 Rule, where most of the time you are following the guidelines defined above, and some of the time you indulge in your cravings. Here are some tips to consider as you embark on this new path ripe with mindful, delicious foods:

**Food preparation**

The energy we infuse our food with is the energy that fuels our body. If we are hurried and rushed while we are cooking, our digestion will be impacted. Preparing your food mindfully means learning to enjoy the process from beginning to end. Try some of the following methods to introduce pleasure into your daily diet:

**Buy local, fresh food**

When shopping, try to choose organic foods whenever possible. Consider what grows from the earth and what will nourish your body. Ideally, we would buy fresh food each day to be cooked that night. If lifestyle permits, buy from your local farmers market or buy local produce.

**Set the scene for pleasurable eating**

So often we eat on the fly, talking on the phone, watching TV, completely distracted. Consider a different experience: set the table for yourself, put on some calming music and light some candles. Be it breakfast, lunch or dinner, treat yourself like royalty and take some time to nourish and relax.

**Bless your meal**

At Thanksgiving, people often say grace, but it is not a common practice in many homes. Taking some time to be grateful for the food on your plate and blessings in your life infuse you with the feelings of love and appreciation, invoking the pleasure feeling. Silent or out loud, a blessing can set the tone for a delicious meal.

**Taste each bite**

Now that you are all set to enjoy your meal, take the time to taste the food. Some recommend up to 30 bites per chew, putting your fork down in between. By liquefying the food in your mouth, the digestion process is improved drastically, and no water is needed to wash down the food.

**Consider your mood**

If you, like most, have a habit of emotional eating, ask yourself what you really need before you dive into the barrel of cookies. Are you feeling low energy? Truly hungry? Thirsty? Sleepy? Stressed? Low on energy? Sometimes, if you take a few moments to check in with yourself, you will realize that what you are really craving is something other than food: time alone, exercise, journaling, social interaction, etc.

## Including Fertile Foods in your daily menu

*Recipes from: Cooking for Fertility: Foods to Nourish Your Fertile Soul*

**Morning ritual**

- Rise, fully rested to meet the day.
- Practice a mindful breathing meditation for 5-10 minutes before leaping out of bed to meet the day.

- Begin with a cup of hot water to cleanse the palette and aid morning digestion (here begins a day of committing to drinking half your body weight in ounces of room temperature water).
- Movement: 30 minutes of exercise (walking, Qi Gong, Yoga)

**Breakfast: Gourmet oatmeal**

Oats add substance to the diet, calming the nervous system and inviting the relaxation response so important to fertility. Walnuts and flaxseed are full of omega-3 fatty acids, and adding dark berries provides antioxidants to nourish blood and support its flow. Oatmeal is a very nutritious breakfast. Slowly simmered in water, oatmeal benefits the reproductive organs and sets the stage for stable blood sugar and energy levels all day.

Serves 2
Cooking time: 20-30 minutes

3 cups water
1 ½ cups rolled oats
¼ cup raisins
½ cup blueberries
2 teaspoons ground flaxseed
¼ cup crushed walnuts
2 tablespoons applesauce (optional)

Bring water to a boil. Add oats and simmer on

medium heat. Once the water evaporates, add raisins and berries. Place in a bowl and top with flaxseed, walnuts, and/or applesauce, if desired.

**Mid-morning snack: Sprouted fertility loaf with nut butter**

*Featured recipe in Cooking for Fertility DVD with Tiffany Pollard and Kathryn Flynn*

Sprouted grains help to reduce inflammation, counteracting the impact of wheat and refined carbohydrates. Sprouts are high in nutrients and help create an optimal environment for conception and implantation. The addition of sprouted pumpkin seeds provides a dose of healthful omega-3 fatty acids and zinc. Red clover contains vitamin B, thiamine, vitamin C, and calcium, which help relax the nervous system and alkalize cervical mucous, creating an ideal PH balance in the uterus. Top with delicious nut butter for a balanced protein-carbohydrate start to the day.

Yields 1 medium loaf
Cooking time: I hour

Sprouting instructions: In two separate bowls, jars or pots soak quinoa and pumpkin seeds overnight; use enough water to cover the grains and seeds by 3 to 4 inches. The next morning drain, rinse with cool water and drain again. Repeat this procedure twice a day, for one to two days until you see sprouts of approximately 1/4 inch.

2 cups quinoa seeds
½ cup pumpkin seeds
¼ cup red clover
1 teaspoon cinnamon
¼ cup apple juice
3 tablespoon agave nectar
2 to 3 tablespoons unrefined olive oil for drizzling on top

Preheat oven to 350 degrees. Combine sprouted seeds, red clover, cinnamon, agave and apple juice in a large bowl. Transfer mixture to a food processor and blend until smooth "dough like" consistency is achieved. Place loaf mixture in a lightly greased loaf pan and bake for approximately 1 hour or more until golden brown on top and cooked through. Try drizzling some unrefined olive oil on top just after it comes out of the oven.

**Nut butter** provides a good source of protein and fat.

2 cups organic nuts (almonds, cashews, hazelnuts, walnuts)
2 tablespoons unrefined sesame oil
Salt to taste

Soak nuts in water overnight. Combine nuts and salt in food processor, chopping until finely ground. Add oil and continue to mix until desired texture.

**Lunch: Fertility stew**

This nourishing soup is created specifically for fertility with purifying garlic and onions, mineral-rich seaweed, cruciferous vegetables, calming brown rice, yams to stimulate the ovaries, and tofu for cooling replenishment. With balanced grains, vegetables and protein, this soup makes a complete meal.

Serves 4
Cooking time: 40 minutes

2 teaspoons extra virgin olive oil
3 cloves garlic, minced
1 Portobello mushroom, sliced thinly
2 leeks, chopped
2 celery stalks
1 small head cabbage
6 plum tomatoes, diced
32 ounces organic chicken or vegetable stock
1 yam, cubed
1 piece dried kelp
1 6-ounce package tofu or 2 cups shrimp
1 cup brown rice, cooked
1/2cup broccoli, chopped
1 cup black beans, cooked

In a large pot heat olive oil, and sauté garlic, mushrooms, leeks, and celery until browned. Add cabbage and tomatoes, simmering for five minutes. Add broth, yam, and kelp. Bring to a boil. After 10 minutes reduce heat, and add tofu or shrimp, black beans, rice, and broccoli. When broccoli becomes bright green, soup is ready.

**Mid-afternoon snack: Hummus and wheat free crackers (rice crackers, Mary's gone crackers)**

**Hummus**

Garbanzo beans contain more iron than any other legume, an important ingredient for building blood if you have heavy periods, which can lead to iron deficiency anemia, or if you have conditions where your bleeding is light in color or scanty. They are also a good source of healthy fats and delicious for spreading on sandwiches and rice crackers.

Yields 2 cups

2 cups garbanzo beans (also called chickpeas)-canned is fine
1 tablespoon tahini (sesame seed paste)
1 tablespoon extra virgin olive oil
Juice of 1/2 a fresh lemon
2 garlic cloves, minced
2 tablespoons fresh cilantro
¼ teaspoon turmeric

Combine garbanzo beans, tahini, olive oil, lemon juice, garlic and cilantro in a food processor. Pulse until smooth. Transfer to a serving bowl, garnish with turmeric and chill.

**Dinner: Poached salmon with pineapple sauce serve with steamed asparagus**

*Featured recipe in Cooking for Fertility DVD with Tiffany Pollard and Kathryn Flynn*

Wild salmon is one of the richest sources of healthful omega-3 fatty acids, known to reduce blood clotting and increase circulation to damaged tissues in the body. It is also an essential component for in-utero brain development of babies. In this recipe, we have added implantation-enhancing bromelain in pineapple. Enjoy salmon several times a week.

Serves 3 to 4
Cooking time: 10 to 12 minutes

Up to 4 cups of organic chicken or veggie broth
1 pound wild salmon fillets
Salt and pepper to taste
Chopped parsley and or red bell pepper for garnish
Optional: 4 pineapple slices set on side of each plate

Pineapple sauce
Yields: 3/4 cup

1/2 cup fresh or frozen pineapple, chopped

2 to 3 Tablespoons agave nectar
2 tablespoons Dijon mustard

Fill a skillet one-third full of broth and put on medium low heat; add salmon and cover (you want for the liquid to be at least half way up on the side of the highest part of the fish fillet). Turn the heat low, so salmon poaches in the broth and steam, until bright pink and easily flaked with a knife (approximately 10-12 minutes). In a blender or food processor, combine pineapple, agave, and mustard. Plate the fish, drizzle with pineapple sauce. Serve with grilled asparagus.

**Evening relaxation ritual**

- Foot soak with Epsom salts
- Chamomile tea with light reading
- Bed before 11pm to promote hormonal balance and aid liver regeneration

# Step 8:
# Trust Nature's Cycle

## The miracle of conception

The process of creating a new life involves a symphony of intricate players that join in concert to produce a living, breathing person. Life requires that the sex cells of a female (egg/ovum) unite with the sex cells of a male (spermatozoa) to create the beginnings of a new life. Consider for a moment all of the events that came into play to produce the outcome of you. First came the chance meeting between your parents who would provide you with a combination of two unique genetic imprints. And then, just imagine the synergy in their union: up to 400 million spermatozoa vying to fertilize your mother's egg and in most cases only one "lucky" sperm triumphs.[xcvi] Consider the possibility that each of those 400 million sperm cells contained a slightly different genetic makeup that influenced the outcome of who you are. Understanding all of the pieces that must come into play for pregnancy to occur illuminates the miracle of life.

As men and women, most of us come into the

world with all that we need to reproduce: basic anatomy, cells, hormones and fluids. Scientists are discovering that the exchange of sex cells between a man and a woman may simply be the beginning of creation. Our physiology creates the opportunity for manifestation, but what role do our minds and spirits play in shaping our outcome? More and more the connections between our minds and bodies are being uncovered, revealing that our emotions and thoughts impact our physical being.

> *Rather than genes "controlling" biology, it is now recognized that environment, and more specifically, our perception of the environment, profoundly influences our structure, behavior and gene activity. An understanding of the newly described cell-control mechanisms will cause as profound a shift in biological belief as the quantum revolution caused in physics. Though mass consciousness is still imbued with the belief that the character of our lives is controlled by genes, a radically new understanding is unfolding at the leading edge of science. The strength in the emerging new biological model is that it unifies the basic philosophies of conventional medicine, Oriental medicine and spiritual healing.*[xcvii]
>
> *—Bruce H. Lipton, Ph.D. 2004*

Sciences grace us with the understanding of how we reproduce, in terms of specific interactions between sex organs, hormones and bodily cycles. Eastern medicine supports the body as a whole, rather than looking only to the individual sex organs for answers to fertility. Through this lens, the body is viewed as a microcosm of nature and the greater universe; what happens in one organ system has a direct impact on all organ systems. When our bodies are in balance with nature and our environment, conception can occur. Beginning with a deep understanding of our body's physiology and nature's cycles, we become the conductors of our own bodily orchestra. Revealing the relationship between our bodies and minds in relationship to the whole, we begin to unveil the secret of our fertility.

## Human Reproduction

Human reproduction has evolved over the years and is regarded as a most rational process, especially when compared to other species on our planet. Consider the haphazard reproduction technique of fish for example: without actual physical contact, the female fish releases her eggs, while the male fish swims overhead and drops his sperm in hopes of fertilization. The anatomy of men (penis) and women (vagina) makes the process much more functional. Furthermore, human beings carry within a desire for pleasure: the libido. A healthy libido reveals our most fertile times through a release of hormones in the male (testes) and female (ovaries) urging us to unite.

## Female Reproductive Anatomy

### Facts:[xcviii]

- 98% of girls menstruate by age 15, typically between the ages of 12 and 13.
- Women generally follow the four-week cycle of the moon from onset of menstruation (menarche) to the time her period stops (menopause).
- Variations in the length of a women's cycle occur most at menarche and menopause.
- A woman's period generally lasts 3-8 days.
- Typical blood loss during one cycle is less than 4 tablespoons.
- A woman carries all the eggs she will ever have in her womb when she is born.

### The core

Inside a women's body multiple processes co-exist to produce the monthly cycle and create opportunities for conception. The organs listed below serve as the foundation for the female reproductive system, detailing how and when menstruation and conception occur.

In Chinese medicine, reproductive function corresponds with the water element, our deepest source energies. At birth the kidneys, adrenals and reproductive organs form together and their health is highly dependent on our ability to nourish our reserves with adequate rest, proper nourishment and by reducing life stressors.

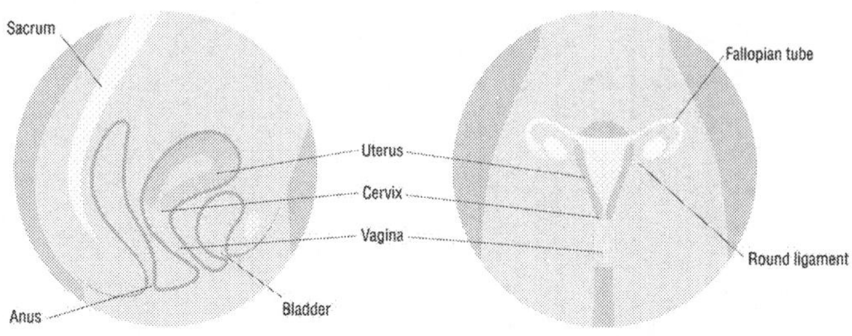


## Ovaries

Most women have a right and a left ovary, though only one is necessary for conception. These grape sized organs produce the ova, or egg cells, that eventually produce one mature ovum each month. The ovaries are endocrine glands, producing estrogen during the first half of the cycle, progesterone during the second half of the cycle and small amounts of testosterone and folliculostatin or inhibin. Most often, the right and the left ovary alternate from month to month, releasing only one mature egg per month. In cases where one ovary has been surgically removed, the remaining ovary takes over and assumes the role of egg maturation and release. When a baby girl is born, she carries all the eggs cells she will have for her entire lifetime.

Dr. Christiane Northrup believes that a woman's ovaries represent her power in the world, much like a man's testicles. In *Women's Bodies, Women's Wisdom*, Dr. Northrup states that, "our ovarian wisdom represents our deepest creativity, that which can be born only through us." She feels "a woman's ovaries are at risk when she feels controlled or criticized by others or when they, themselves, control and criticize others."[xcix]

**Fallopian tubes**

The fallopian tubes frame the uterus and act as the conduit to carry the egg from the ovary to the uterus. The fallopian tubes resemble a cornucopia with fingerlike fimbria, reaching toward the ovary at ovulation in hopes of obtaining the matured ovum. Fallopian tubes are lined with cilia, tiny hair like projections that help to encourage the egg through the tube and toward the womb. During ovulation, secretions increase producing a smooth, slippery procession for the egg to reach the uterus.

Dr. Randine Lewis paints a picture of fallopian tubes as fully conscious organisms with an innate intelligence to maximize opportunities for conception. Cases exist where a woman with only a left ovary and a right fallopian tube is able to conceive, because the fingerlike fimbria at the top of the fallopian tube reached over to the opposite side and grabbed the mature egg, illuminating the fallopian tube as an intentional, opportunity creating sex organ.[c]

**Uterus**

The eventual womb for the fertilized egg, the uterus, contains the endometrial lining, which thickens throughout the month to house the potential of implantation. The uterus is shaped and sized like a pear, weighing a mere 2-3 ounces. The uterus is divided into two parts: the corpus (upper portion) which provides the opening for the egg and the cervix (lower portion) which will be the eventual passageway for the baby. When the egg has not been fertilized, the uterus sheds its lining through the process of menstruation.

"Think of the uterus as the rich dark earth in which the creative seeds from the ovaries grow in time. Our uterus", Northrup says, "is energetically related to our innermost sense of self, symbolic of our dreams, the parts of us we would like to give birth to. Its state of health reflects her inner emotional reality and her belief in herself at the deepest level. The health of the uterus is at risk if a woman doesn't believe in herself or is excessively self-critical."[ci]

### Vagina

The vagina is the narrow passageway at the end of the uterus that leads to the outside of the body. The vagina is the receptive organ through which conception is realized by allowing a man's penis to enter. It is also the eventual birth canal and the avenue from which menstrual blood leaves the body.

The first chakra houses our sense of security in the world. Signified by the color red, our foundational chakra encompasses our ideologies of sex, security and family. Vaginal expression can be strengthened using "kegals" and by learning about what brings us pleasure.

## A woman's natural cycle

Women have for a long time been connected with the ebb and flow of the tides and the waxing and waning of the moon. In ancient times, a woman's body was so in tune with her natural surroundings that women would ovulate and menstruate in groups. Physically, our bodies mirror the cycles of nature through several different processes that set the stage for menstruation, ovulation and conception. The elegant interplay of a woman's cycle illuminates the synergistic connection between all things internal and external in the creation of life.

**The hormonal cycle:** the ebb and flow of substances and secretions produced our hormones; the chemical messengers that govern the entire reproductive process.

**The endometrial cycle:** the rise and fall of the uterine lining to prepare for the fertilized egg. Without implantation, the lining is released during the menstrual cycle.

**The ovarian cycle:** the development and expression of the egg cell through maturation to its journey from the fallopian tube, where it meets sperm and has the opportunity to implant.

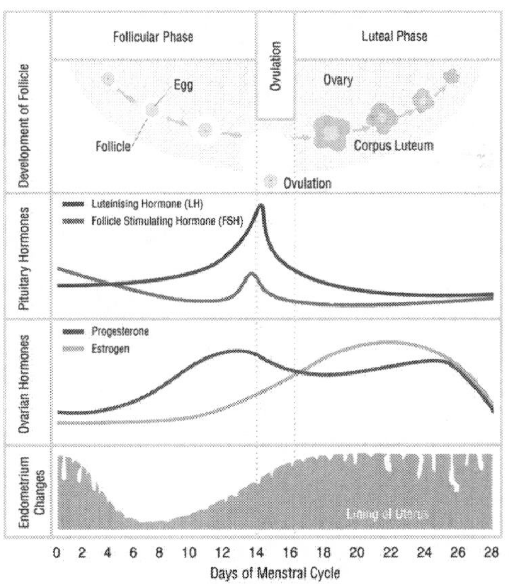

## The Conductors of our Hormonal Cycle

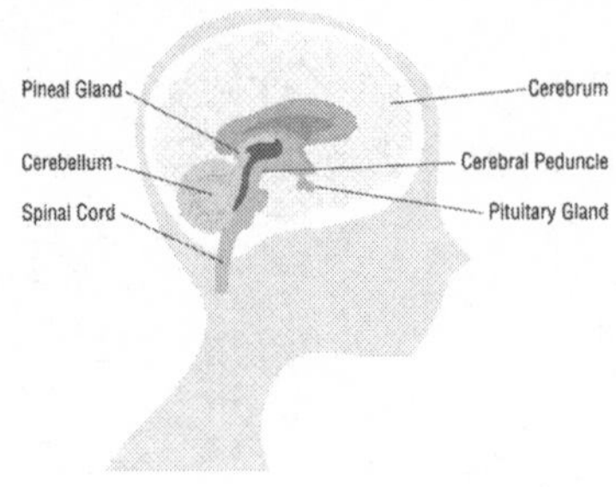


Healthy communication between the brain and the reproductive system is essential. The Hypothalamus-Pituitary-Adrenal (HPA) axis governs the hormones as well as the stress reaction in our body. Chronic perceived stress inhibits the HPA's ability to function properly, compromising the endocrine system as well as immunity.

The hypothalamus lives at the base of the brain and creates the Gonatropin releasing hormone (GnRH), stimulating the pituitary gland to release hormones called gonatropins, thereby triggering egg follicles to develop in the ovary in preparation for ovulation and eventual fertilization and implantation.

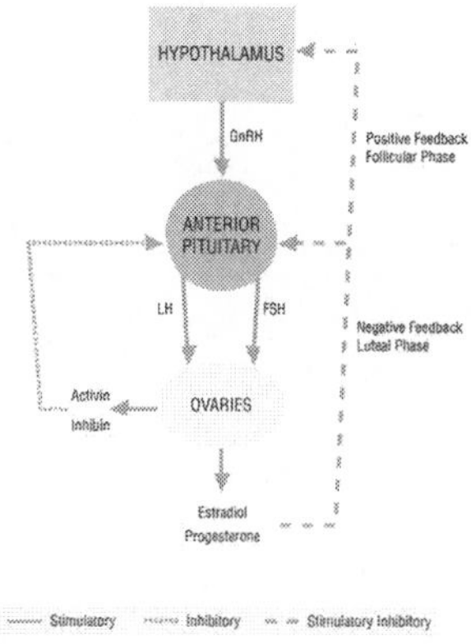


## The pituitary gland releases gonadotropins[cii]

**Follicle stimulating hormone** (FSH) is produced by the pituitary gland and stimulates growth of follicles in the ovaries, which secrete estrogen.

**Luteinizing hormone** (LH) is also produced by pituitary gland. LH works in concert with FSH to trigger ovulation and the release of estrogen and progesterone.

**Prolactin** impacts the ovary's response to FSH and LH as well as the maturation of the follicle and corpus luteum.

## The Endometrial Cycle

The menstrual phase begins on the first day of a woman's period and involves the shedding of the uterine lining. When implantation has not occurred, production of the corpus luteum slows, and progesterone and estrogen secretions lessen. This drop in hormones signals the uterine lining to release blood, cells and tissue to be replenished in the following cycle. The menstrual phase illuminates the uterus as a unique organ in its capacity to shed and renew each cycle.

The proliferative phase begins at the end of menstruation. As the ovarian follicle matures and releases estrogen, the endometrium replenishes and begins to thicken. The endometrium has the potential to thicken from .5 to 5.0 inches during days 7-21, creating a healthy lining for implantation.

During the secretory phase, the corpus luteum (formed by the follicle from which the dominant egg was released) releases additional progesterone. During this phase, the endometrium stops thickening and begins to secrete fluids rich in glycogens (sugar) from open blood vessels and glands (as many as 15 000 glands open during the secretory phase).

## The Ovarian Cycle

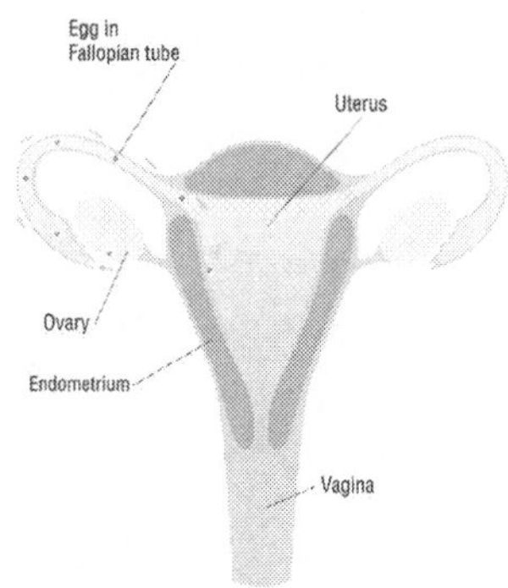


**The ovaries and corpus luteum secrete:**

- **Estrogen** helps to build the uterine wall for implantation, assists in the egg maturation process and provides feedback to inhibit FSH and increase LH.
- **Progesterone** stimulates thickening of the uterine wall and supports implantation.

**The Follicular Phase:** begins with the release of FSH from the pituitary gland, under the influence of GnRH. During this time, some of the follicles in a woman's ovary begin to develop a fluid, and some randomly continue to grow larger than others. Follicles that do not develop simply disappear. The follicular phase follows the same cycle as the menstrual and proliferative phase.

**The Ovulatory Phase:** Once the follicle reaches a

certain stage of development, LH is released by the pituitary gland. Mid-cycle, ovulation occurs when LH surges in concert with estrogen secretions and releases the dominant egg to be gathered by the fallopian tube. Women generally ovulate 14-16 days before their next period.

**The Luteal Phase:** After ovulation, the follicle left over from the dominant egg becomes the corpus luteum and begins more progesterone with small amounts of estrogen. In the case that pregnancy occurs, the corpus luteum will continue to release progesterone to support implantation. If the egg has not been fertilized, progesterone production drops, and the menstrual flow begins. The Luteal phase lasts anywhere between 12-16 days and follows the same timeline as the secretory phase of the endometrial cycle.

**A day-by-day guide to the cycle of menstruation and conception**

** It is important to note that menstrual cycles vary in length and we are using 28 days not as the "norm" but for the simplicity of the explanation.*

**Days 1-3:** The brain and ovary receive hormones released by pituitary gland, signaling follicles in the right or left ovary to begin maturing.

**Days 6-13:** After menstruation, our bodies select the dominant egg that has matured from the follicles. Estrogen encourages the endometrium to begin thickening and will continue throughout the menstrual cycle for possible implantation.

**Day 14 - Ovulation:** A surge of hormones causes the dominant mature egg to be released from the ovary.

**Days 15-25:** The mature egg travels through the fallopian, guided by small hair-like "cilia" that assist the egg to its final destination: the uterus. At the same time, the now-empty follicle transforms into the corpus luteum, which produces progesterone, along with some estrogen, in preparation for implantation of the fertilized egg.

**Days 25-28:** The possibility of implantation is realized, and if it has not occurred, the corpus luteum disintegrates and estrogen and progesterone levels fall, causing the endometrium to break down. The result is shedding of the endometrium through menstruation, which begins day 1 of the cycle again.

## Charting your cycle with nature's rhythm

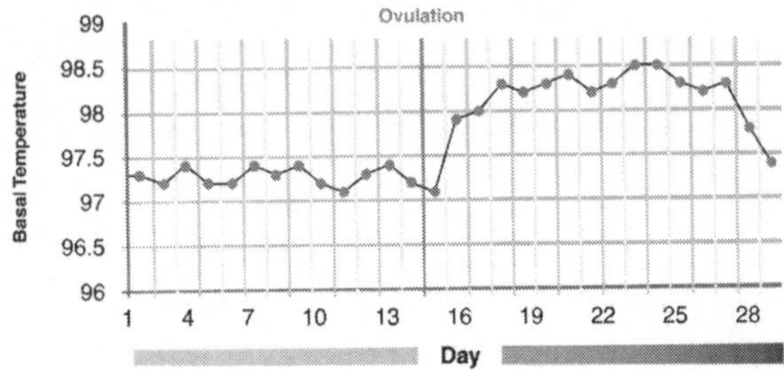


To observe the full elegance of nature in your own monthly cycles is nothing short of empowering. By looking at the subtle changes that occur through the different phases of your cycle, you can begin to address fertility signs and promote balance in your body. By noting the ebbs and flows of your body's cyclical nature, you can determine the first day of your cycle, your waking temperature and changes in your cervical fluid, which unveil your most fertile days, while establishing a full understanding of your unique cycle. In *The Fertile Secret*, we will give you a brief overview of charting your cycle, however it is highly recommended that you read *Taking Charge of Your Fertility* by Toni Weschler to get a full and complete understanding for how to chart your cycle to optimize your fertility.

## Learning How to Chart Your Cycle[ciii]

Photocopy several months worth of Body Basal Temperature (BBT) charts. Follow the three steps below, entering your information each day to track your cycles. What do you notice? PMS? Scant cervical fluid? Heavy or scant menstrual blood? Long or short menstrual cycles? Take note: all of these signs are indicators of your fertility and ability to conceive in a given cycle.

**Basal Body Temperature Chart** Month: ............ Cycle: ............

| Cycle Day | 1 | 2 | 3 | 4 | 5 | 6 | 7 | 8 | 9 | 10 | 11 | 12 | 13 | 14 | 15 | 16 | 17 | 18 | 19 | 20 | 21 | 22 | 23 | 24 | 25 | 26 | 27 | 28 | 29 | 30 | 31 | 32 | 33 | 34 | 35 | 36 | 37 | 38 | 39 | 40 |
|---|---|---|---|---|---|---|---|---|---|---|---|---|---|---|---|---|---|---|---|---|---|---|---|---|---|---|---|---|---|---|---|---|---|---|---|---|---|---|---|---|
| Day of Week | | | | | | | | | | | | | | | | | | | | | | | | | | | | | | | | | | | | | | | | |
| Time | | | | | | | | | | | | | | | | | | | | | | | | | | | | | | | | | | | | | | | | |
| Waking Basal Temp | 99 | 99 | 99 | 99 | 99 | 99 | 99 | 99 | 99 | 99 | 99 | 99 | 99 | 99 | 99 | 99 | 99 | 99 | 99 | 99 | 99 | 99 | 99 | 99 | 99 | 99 | 99 | 99 | 99 | 99 | 99 | 99 | 99 | 99 | 99 | 99 | 99 | 99 | 99 | 99 |
| | 9 | 9 | 9 | 9 | 9 | 9 | 9 | 9 | 9 | 9 | 9 | 9 | 9 | 9 | 9 | 9 | 9 | 9 | 9 | 9 | 9 | 9 | 9 | 9 | 9 | 9 | 9 | 9 | 9 | 9 | 9 | 9 | 9 | 9 | 9 | 9 | 9 | 9 | 9 | 9 |
| | 8 | 8 | 8 | 8 | 8 | 8 | 8 | 8 | 8 | 8 | 8 | 8 | 8 | 8 | 8 | 8 | 8 | 8 | 8 | 8 | 8 | 8 | 8 | 8 | 8 | 8 | 8 | 8 | 8 | 8 | 8 | 8 | 8 | 8 | 8 | 8 | 8 | 8 | 8 | 8 |
| | 7 | 7 | 7 | 7 | 7 | 7 | 7 | 7 | 7 | 7 | 7 | 7 | 7 | 7 | 7 | 7 | 7 | 7 | 7 | 7 | 7 | 7 | 7 | 7 | 7 | 7 | 7 | 7 | 7 | 7 | 7 | 7 | 7 | 7 | 7 | 7 | 7 | 7 | 7 | 7 |
| | 6 | 6 | 6 | 6 | 6 | 6 | 6 | 6 | 6 | 6 | 6 | 6 | 6 | 6 | 6 | 6 | 6 | 6 | 6 | 6 | 6 | 6 | 6 | 6 | 6 | 6 | 6 | 6 | 6 | 6 | 6 | 6 | 6 | 6 | 6 | 6 | 6 | 6 | 6 | 6 |
| | 5 | 5 | 5 | 5 | 5 | 5 | 5 | 5 | 5 | 5 | 5 | 5 | 5 | 5 | 5 | 5 | 5 | 5 | 5 | 5 | 5 | 5 | 5 | 5 | 5 | 5 | 5 | 5 | 5 | 5 | 5 | 5 | 5 | 5 | 5 | 5 | 5 | 5 | 5 | 5 |
| | 4 | 4 | 4 | 4 | 4 | 4 | 4 | 4 | 4 | 4 | 4 | 4 | 4 | 4 | 4 | 4 | 4 | 4 | 4 | 4 | 4 | 4 | 4 | 4 | 4 | 4 | 4 | 4 | 4 | 4 | 4 | 4 | 4 | 4 | 4 | 4 | 4 | 4 | 4 | 4 |
| | 3 | 3 | 3 | 3 | 3 | 3 | 3 | 3 | 3 | 3 | 3 | 3 | 3 | 3 | 3 | 3 | 3 | 3 | 3 | 3 | 3 | 3 | 3 | 3 | 3 | 3 | 3 | 3 | 3 | 3 | 3 | 3 | 3 | 3 | 3 | 3 | 3 | 3 | 3 | 3 |
| | 2 | 2 | 2 | 2 | 2 | 2 | 2 | 2 | 2 | 2 | 2 | 2 | 2 | 2 | 2 | 2 | 2 | 2 | 2 | 2 | 2 | 2 | 2 | 2 | 2 | 2 | 2 | 2 | 2 | 2 | 2 | 2 | 2 | 2 | 2 | 2 | 2 | 2 | 2 | 2 |
| | 1 | 1 | 1 | 1 | 1 | 1 | 1 | 1 | 1 | 1 | 1 | 1 | 1 | 1 | 1 | 1 | 1 | 1 | 1 | 1 | 1 | 1 | 1 | 1 | 1 | 1 | 1 | 1 | 1 | 1 | 1 | 1 | 1 | 1 | 1 | 1 | 1 | 1 | 1 | 1 |
| | 98 | 98 | 98 | 98 | 98 | 98 | 98 | 98 | 98 | 98 | 98 | 98 | 98 | 98 | 98 | 98 | 98 | 98 | 98 | 98 | 98 | 98 | 98 | 98 | 98 | 98 | 98 | 98 | 98 | 98 | 98 | 98 | 98 | 98 | 98 | 98 | 98 | 98 | 98 | 98 |
| | 9 | 9 | 9 | 9 | 9 | 9 | 9 | 9 | 9 | 9 | 9 | 9 | 9 | 9 | 9 | 9 | 9 | 9 | 9 | 9 | 9 | 9 | 9 | 9 | 9 | 9 | 9 | 9 | 9 | 9 | 9 | 9 | 9 | 9 | 9 | 9 | 9 | 9 | 9 | 9 |
| | 8 | 8 | 8 | 8 | 8 | 8 | 8 | 8 | 8 | 8 | 8 | 8 | 8 | 8 | 8 | 8 | 8 | 8 | 8 | 8 | 8 | 8 | 8 | 8 | 8 | 8 | 8 | 8 | 8 | 8 | 8 | 8 | 8 | 8 | 8 | 8 | 8 | 8 | 8 | 8 |
| | 7 | 7 | 7 | 7 | 7 | 7 | 7 | 7 | 7 | 7 | 7 | 7 | 7 | 7 | 7 | 7 | 7 | 7 | 7 | 7 | 7 | 7 | 7 | 7 | 7 | 7 | 7 | 7 | 7 | 7 | 7 | 7 | 7 | 7 | 7 | 7 | 7 | 7 | 7 | 7 |
| | 6 | 6 | 6 | 6 | 6 | 6 | 6 | 6 | 6 | 6 | 6 | 6 | 6 | 6 | 6 | 6 | 6 | 6 | 6 | 6 | 6 | 6 | 6 | 6 | 6 | 6 | 6 | 6 | 6 | 6 | 6 | 6 | 6 | 6 | 6 | 6 | 6 | 6 | 6 | 6 |
| | 5 | 5 | 5 | 5 | 5 | 5 | 5 | 5 | 5 | 5 | 5 | 5 | 5 | 5 | 5 | 5 | 5 | 5 | 5 | 5 | 5 | 5 | 5 | 5 | 5 | 5 | 5 | 5 | 5 | 5 | 5 | 5 | 5 | 5 | 5 | 5 | 5 | 5 | 5 | 5 |
| | 4 | 4 | 4 | 4 | 4 | 4 | 4 | 4 | 4 | 4 | 4 | 4 | 4 | 4 | 4 | 4 | 4 | 4 | 4 | 4 | 4 | 4 | 4 | 4 | 4 | 4 | 4 | 4 | 4 | 4 | 4 | 4 | 4 | 4 | 4 | 4 | 4 | 4 | 4 | 4 |
| | 3 | 3 | 3 | 3 | 3 | 3 | 3 | 3 | 3 | 3 | 3 | 3 | 3 | 3 | 3 | 3 | 3 | 3 | 3 | 3 | 3 | 3 | 3 | 3 | 3 | 3 | 3 | 3 | 3 | 3 | 3 | 3 | 3 | 3 | 3 | 3 | 3 | 3 | 3 | 3 |
| | 2 | 2 | 2 | 2 | 2 | 2 | 2 | 2 | 2 | 2 | 2 | 2 | 2 | 2 | 2 | 2 | 2 | 2 | 2 | 2 | 2 | 2 | 2 | 2 | 2 | 2 | 2 | 2 | 2 | 2 | 2 | 2 | 2 | 2 | 2 | 2 | 2 | 2 | 2 | 2 |
| | 1 | 1 | 1 | 1 | 1 | 1 | 1 | 1 | 1 | 1 | 1 | 1 | 1 | 1 | 1 | 1 | 1 | 1 | 1 | 1 | 1 | 1 | 1 | 1 | 1 | 1 | 1 | 1 | 1 | 1 | 1 | 1 | 1 | 1 | 1 | 1 | 1 | 1 | 1 | 1 |
| | 97 | 97 | 97 | 97 | 97 | 97 | 97 | 97 | 97 | 97 | 97 | 97 | 97 | 97 | 97 | 97 | 97 | 97 | 97 | 97 | 97 | 97 | 97 | 97 | 97 | 97 | 97 | 97 | 97 | 97 | 97 | 97 | 97 | 97 | 97 | 97 | 97 | 97 | 97 | 97 |
| | 9 | 9 | 9 | 9 | 9 | 9 | 9 | 9 | 9 | 9 | 9 | 9 | 9 | 9 | 9 | 9 | 9 | 9 | 9 | 9 | 9 | 9 | 9 | 9 | 9 | 9 | 9 | 9 | 9 | 9 | 9 | 9 | 9 | 9 | 9 | 9 | 9 | 9 | 9 | 9 |
| | 8 | 8 | 8 | 8 | 8 | 8 | 8 | 8 | 8 | 8 | 8 | 8 | 8 | 8 | 8 | 8 | 8 | 8 | 8 | 8 | 8 | 8 | 8 | 8 | 8 | 8 | 8 | 8 | 8 | 8 | 8 | 8 | 8 | 8 | 8 | 8 | 8 | 8 | 8 | 8 |
| **Cycle Day** | 1 | 2 | 3 | 4 | 5 | 6 | 7 | 8 | 9 | 10 | 11 | 12 | 13 | 14 | 15 | 16 | 17 | 18 | 19 | 20 | 21 | 22 | 23 | 24 | 25 | 26 | 27 | 28 | 29 | 30 | 31 | 32 | 33 | 34 | 35 | 36 | 37 | 38 | 39 | 40 |
| Circle Day of Intercourse | | | | | | | | | | | | | | | | | | | | | | | | | | | | | | | | | | | | | | | | |
| Describe Cervical Fluid | | | | | | | | | | | | | | | | | | | | | | | | | | | | | | | | | | | | | | | | |
| Cervix Hard/Soft | | | | | | | | | | | | | | | | | | | | | | | | | | | | | | | | | | | | | | | | |
| Cervix Position | | | | | | | | | | | | | | | | | | | | | | | | | | | | | | | | | | | | | | | | |
| Vaginal Sensation | | | | | | | | | | | | | | | | | | | | | | | | | | | | | | | | | | | | | | | | |
| **Cycle Day** | 1 | 2 | 3 | 4 | 5 | 6 | 7 | 8 | 9 | 10 | 11 | 12 | 13 | 14 | 15 | 16 | 17 | 18 | 19 | 20 | 21 | 22 | 23 | 24 | 25 | 26 | 27 | 28 | 29 | 30 | 31 | 32 | 33 | 34 | 35 | 36 | 37 | 38 | 39 | 40 |
| OPK Result | | | | | | | | | | | | | | | | | | | | | | | | | | | | | | | | | | | | | | | | |
| Pregnancy Test Results | | | | | | | | | | | | | | | | | | | | | | | | | | | | | | | | | | | | | | | | |
| Other Notes: | | | | | | | | | | | | | | | | | | | | | | | | | | | | | | | | | | | | | | | | |
| Poor Sleep | | | | | | | | | | | | | | | | | | | | | | | | | | | | | | | | | | | | | | | | |
| Alcohol | | | | | | | | | | | | | | | | | | | | | | | | | | | | | | | | | | | | | | | | |
| Illness | | | | | | | | | | | | | | | | | | | | | | | | | | | | | | | | | | | | | | | | |
| Additional Information | | | | | | | | | | | | | | | | | | | | | | | | | | | | | | | | | | | | | | | | |

| Describe Cervical Fluid | S = Sticky C = Creamy E = Eggwhite | Cervix Hard/Soft | S = Soft H = Hard | Cervix Position | L = Low M = Middle H = High | Vaginal Sensation | D = Dry M = Moist W = Wet |
|---|---|---|---|---|---|---|---|

**1. The onset of menstruation:** your first day of bleeding is considered Day 1 on your chart. The shedding of the endometrium lining, shows that a pregnancy has not occurred during the previous month and therefore marks the beginning of your follicular phase (the pre-ovulatory phase of your cycle).

**2. Cervical fluid:** as ovulation approaches, estrogen levels begin to rise, causing your cervix to secrete a substance that acts as a conduit to help the sperm swim up to fertilize the egg in the fallopian tubes. After conception, the fertilized egg will travel down to the uterus and implant.

In Toni Weschler's, *Taking Charge of Your Fertility*, she discusses a continuum of cervical fluid on the road to ovulation including:[civ]

- Sticky: not overly conducive to fertility
- Creamy: may support the life of the sperm
- Wet: the most fertile, often resembling egg white in consistency

**3. Your waking temperature:** first thing in the morning, before you even get out of bed, take your body's resting (basal body) temperature with a basal thermometer and circle it on your chart. Try to take it about the same time every morning, give or take an hour or so. A shift in temperature at least 0.2° Fahrenheit higher than the highest of the last 6 temperatures indicates that ovulation may have occurred. If you are pregnant your temperature will remain elevated at least 18 days.

# Step 9: Appreciate the Advances of Western Medicine

## The Diagnostic Process

In the last decades, amazing advances have been made in the field of reproductive medicine, allowing men and women previously diagnosed "infertile" to conceive. Advanced research in the medical field has introduced new diagnostic tools, ovulatory medications and fertility procedures that have opened a world of possibilities to scenarios that once seemed hopeless. Geneticists have created avenues to predetermine the outcome of a healthy fetus. And yet, the interesting thing about western medicine is that we are still learning. Many processes of the human reproductive system remain somewhat of a mystery, and while hormone panels and ultrasounds give us helpful information, the reason why women with similar diagnoses end up with different outcomes is puzzling at times.

Perhaps one of the most forward-thinking elements of Western medicine is its rather new consideration of complementary medicine, and the role of the mind with the body in determining the outcome of diagnoses. How does thought and intention impact our diagnoses? In my own practice, I have noticed that how I engage with a client can impact their experience. Consider for a moment the level of trust one puts in the doctor to tell one what is right and wrong in terms of how one's body is working. So many of the words we use in fertility start off on the wrong foot. How does a woman feel when she hears the diagnosis of "old eggs," "poor ovarian responder," or "blocked tubes?" There is an element of saying it like it is in medicine, but do we stop to think how our words might be impacting the outcome?

What if, instead, we began to focus on the possibility of a given scenario? Knowing that all we can do is move forward and do the things within our ability, why not look at each case through the lens of hope and possibility and walk through the journey with an open mind. In *My Stroke of Insight*, Dr. Jill Bolton Taylor explains to us why client care just may be the most important part of any healing journey. As a brain doctor, she woke up one morning and consciously observed the process of losing the functioning of her body to a stroke. During her long recovery, she experienced an energetic connection to those who were caring for her, definitively noting that how each caregiver approached her mattered the most. Those who came gently and kindly towards her gave her energy and the will to recover; those who were rough, abrupt and hurried stole energy.[cv] I agree wholeheartedly with her statement. How we interact with clients in our care matters. My own personal experience of caring for my mother through her recent stroke reaffirmed my belief: love and kindness heal.

The diagnostic process involves numerous tests, but there is no reason to create fear around the process. Remember, diagnoses are not static; fertility is an evolutionary process where things change and there are no absolutes. What matters the most is that the physician and the client are in a partnership to produce great health. This section details the process of discovery through intake, testing and options for treatment with the intention of clarifying what to expect, and removing any fear of the unknown.

## A. The intake

When looking for the cause of reproductive dysfunction, it is essential to meet with the couple for the health history and physical examination. Often times, society thinks of infertility as a "female" issue. The truth is that as much as 50% of reproductive issues stem from a man's fertility. By meeting with the couple together, we are able to get a more accurate picture of the couple's fertility prognosis and develop a fully supportive protocol.

## Health History

### 1. Sexual Habits: frequency of intercourse, length of time "trying to conceive"

The evaluation begins with a health history. A couple that comes to a reproductive endocrinologist has generally been trying to conceive for a year regularly, without contraception. What is interesting is that when you probe a little deeper, couples often reveal that though they were not "trying," they have been sexually active without contraception for much longer without becoming pregnant.

Another scenario may be that sexual intercourse has not been regular or frequent enough to create the opportunity for pregnancy. The longer a couple has in fact been attempting to conceive without pregnancy, the more likely it is that we will find a factor in our exam that indicates a cause of infertility. Conversely, a diagnosis is considerably less likely with a shorter window of trying to conceive. With regards to a couple's sexual habits we also ask the following:

For the woman:

- Pelvic pain before, during, or after intercourse?
- Vaginal dryness?
- Ability to achieve orgasm?

For the man:

- Pelvic pain?
- Difficulty with erections?
- Does ejaculate occur inter-vaginally?
- Any other children (this is also important early on, even if the man has fathered children, because things can change)?

| Chance of Pregnancy by Day of Intercourse<br>day zero is ovulation | | | | | | | | |
|---|---|---|---|---|---|---|---|---|
| -5 | -4 | -3 | -2 | -1 | 0 | 1 | 2 | 3 |
| 0% | 11% | 15% | 20% | 26% | 15% | 9% | 5% | 0% |

## 2. Age

When choosing a treatment protocol, we consider both how long a couple has been trying to conceive as well as the woman's age. As women enter their mid to late thirties and forties, the chances of conception decrease and we tailor our protocol accordingly. A couple is encouraged to seek help from a reproductive endocrinologist after a year of unprotected sex without conception at age 35, or six months at age 40. Couples are advised to come for an evaluation as early as three months in the case of absent periods, tubal pregnancies or testicular problems in the man. Though the age of the man may not seem as relevant, sexual function and decreased sexual activity can impact chances of pregnancy.

### 3. Cycle regularity: assessing hormonal balance and ovulation patterns

Whether a woman is experiencing regular 28 days cycles will give a good indication as to whether or not she is ovulating. Women often track their cycles by:

1. Charting their body basal temperatures each morning before rising to confirm the 0.4 to 1.0 degree Fahrenheit temperature increase associated with ovulation.
2. Tracking cervical mucous changes throughout the month to reveal the ovulatory phase by noting the variations of wet, stretchy, and slippery mucus.
3. Using ovulation predictor kits to look for the LH rise at ovulation.

Though these are all great tools, the only true proof of ovulation is a pregnancy. While the mechanical processes of ovulation are well explained, the reasons why the mechanism shuts down remain somewhat of a mystery. A woman can stop ovulating due to hormonal miscommunications between the pituitary gland and the hypothalamus, along with diet, stress and other drugs. We do know that endocrine abnormalities like hyper or hypo thyroid, high prolactin and PCOS can all impact ovulation patterns, but are still unable to formally pinpoint the exact way in which it occurs.

### 4. History of live births, miscarriages and abortions

History of prior pregnancies, miscarriages and abortions generally do not seem to effect the risk of infertility, unless it has been associated with an infection, laceration, uterine injury or hemorrhaging resulting from surgeries, including cesareans and full or partial hysterectomies. Any problems associated with delivery can result in emotional trauma and stress that might impact future fertility outcomes.

### 5. Infections and sexually transmitted diseases

Pelvic inflammatory disease (PID) is a major cause of female infertility. PID is comprised of a number of different factors that cause infection in the pelvic region: reproductive organs, appendix, intestine and, most commonly, the fallopian tubes (also salpingtis). Symptoms of PID may include "chills," fever, inflammation and pelvic pain, though in some cases there are no symptoms at all. Frequent, more intense infections increase the chances of scarring, and 20% of women experience an increased risk of ectopic pregnancy and infertility as a result of PID. Some of the most common causes for PID are:

- Multiple sexual partners
- Sexually transmitted diseases: chlamydia trachomatis, gonorrhea and HPV (damages the cervix)
- Surgeries including cesareans or non-sterile abortions
- Pelvic tuberculosis
- Herpes Virus
- Ruptured Appendix

**6. History of illness and disease**

There are a handful of diseases and illness that can lead to infertility in men and women including:

- Toxoplasmosis
- Malaria
- Leprosy
- Tuberculosis
- Mumps
- Sickle Cell Disease
- Cancer with radiation and chemotherapy
- History of orchitis or epididymitis in men (swelling of the testicle or epididymis or coiled tube at back of testicle)
- Mumps (men)
- Varicocele (men)
- Exposure to DES (synthetic estrogen) in the womb distributed from 1938 to 1971 and

believed to prevent miscarriage

- Chronic long-term diseases like diabetes, kidney disease
- Delayed menstruation/puberty
- Autoimmune Disorders
- Reproductive disorders like cervical obstructions, fibroids, endometriosis

**7. Weight, exercise and history of eating disorders**

Since hormones are stored in fat cells, being under or overweight can impact hormonal balance and therefore ovulation. As an indicator of healthy weight, we often look to the body mass index as a tool to classify a person's weight as underweight, average, overweight or obese. What is most encouraging is that no matter where we are today, we each have the power to create a normal BMI (between 19-24) through regular exercise and healthy eating habits.

Eating disorders in particular can prove particularly challenging for fertility. In fact, two of the most common disorders, anorexia and bulimia, have been linked to functional hypothalamic amenorrhea (FHA): the absence of menstruation due to miscommunication between the thyroid gland and the hypothalamus- pituitary adrenal system. In one study, 17% of women treated for infertility had eating disorders.[cvi]

Weight in Pounds

| Height in Feet and Inches | 100 | 110 | 120 | 130 | 140 | 150 | 160 | 170 | 180 | 190 | 200 | 210 | 220 | 230 | 240 | 250 |
|---|---|---|---|---|---|---|---|---|---|---|---|---|---|---|---|---|
| 4' | 30.5 | 33.6 | 36.6 | 39.7 | 42.7 | 45.8 | 48.8 | 51.9 | 54.9 | 58.0 | 61.0 | 64.1 | 67.1 | 70.2 | 73.2 | 76.3 |
| 4'2" | 28.1 | 30.9 | 33.7 | 36.6 | 39.4 | 42.2 | 45.0 | 47.8 | 50.6 | 53.4 | 56.2 | 59.1 | 61.9 | 64.7 | 67.5 | 70.3 |
| 4'4" | 26.0 | 28.6 | 31.2 | 33.8 | 36.4 | 39.0 | 41.6 | 44.2 | 46.8 | 49.4 | 52.0 | 54.6 | 57.2 | 59.8 | 62.4 | 65.0 |
| 4'6" | 24.1 | 26.5 | 28.9 | 31.3 | 33.8 | 36.2 | 38.6 | 41.0 | 43.4 | 45.8 | 48.2 | 50.6 | 53.0 | 55.4 | 57.9 | 60.3 |
| 4'8" | 22.4 | 24.7 | 26.9 | 29.1 | 31.4 | 33.6 | 35.9 | 38.1 | 40.4 | 42.6 | 44.8 | 47.1 | 49.3 | 51.6 | 53.8 | 56.0 |
| 4'10" | 20.9 | 23.0 | 25.1 | 27.2 | 29.3 | 31.3 | 33.4 | 35.5 | 37.6 | 39.7 | 41.8 | 43.9 | 46.0 | 48.1 | 50.2 | 52.2 |
| 5' | 19.5 | 21.5 | 23.4 | 25.4 | 27.3 | 29.3 | 31.2 | 33.2 | 35.2 | 37.1 | 39.1 | 41.0 | 43.0 | 44.9 | 46.9 | 48.8 |
| 5'2" | 18.3 | 20.1 | 21.9 | 23.8 | 25.6 | 27.4 | 29.3 | 31.1 | 32.9 | 34.7 | 36.6 | 38.4 | 40.2 | 42.1 | 43.9 | 45.7 |
| 5'4" | 17.2 | 18.9 | 20.6 | 22.3 | 24.0 | 25.7 | 27.5 | 29.2 | 30.9 | 32.6 | 34.3 | 36.0 | 37.8 | 39.5 | 41.2 | 42.9 |
| 5'6" | 16.1 | 17.8 | 19.4 | 21.0 | 22.6 | 24.2 | 25.8 | 27.4 | 29.0 | 30.7 | 32.3 | 33.9 | 35.5 | 37.1 | 38.7 | 40.3 |
| 5'8" | 15.2 | 16.7 | 18.2 | 19.8 | 21.3 | 22.8 | 24.3 | 25.8 | 27.4 | 28.9 | 30.4 | 31.9 | 33.4 | 35.0 | 36.5 | 38.0 |
| 5'10" | 14.3 | 15.8 | 17.2 | 18.7 | 20.1 | 21.5 | 23.0 | 24.4 | 25.8 | 27.3 | 28.7 | 30.1 | 31.6 | 33.0 | 34.4 | 35.9 |
| 6' | 13.6 | 14.9 | 16.3 | 17.6 | 19.0 | 20.3 | 21.7 | 23.1 | 24.4 | 25.8 | 27.1 | 28.5 | 29.8 | 31.2 | 32.5 | 33.9 |
| 6'2" | 12.8 | 14.1 | 15.4 | 16.7 | 18.0 | 19.3 | 20.5 | 21.8 | 23.1 | 24.4 | 25.7 | 27.0 | 28.2 | 29.5 | 30.8 | 32.1 |
| 6'4" | 12.2 | 13.4 | 14.6 | 15.8 | 17.0 | 18.3 | 19.5 | 20.7 | 21.9 | 23.1 | 24.3 | 25.6 | 26.8 | 28.0 | 29.2 | 30.4 |
| 6'6" | 11.6 | 12.7 | 13.9 | 15.0 | 16.2 | 17.3 | 18.5 | 19.6 | 20.8 | 22.0 | 23.1 | 24.3 | 25.4 | 26.6 | 27.7 | 28.9 |
| 6'8" | 11.0 | 12.1 | 13.2 | 14.3 | 15.4 | 16.5 | 17.6 | 18.7 | 19.8 | 20.9 | 22.0 | 23.1 | 24.2 | 25.3 | 26.4 | 27.5 |
| 6'10" | 10.5 | 11.5 | 12.5 | 13.6 | 14.6 | 15.7 | 16.7 | 17.8 | 18.8 | 19.9 | 20.9 | 22.0 | 23.0 | 24.0 | 25.1 | 26.1 |
| 7' | 10.0 | 11.0 | 12.0 | 13.0 | 13.9 | 14.9 | 15.9 | 16.9 | 17.9 | 18.9 | 19.9 | 20.9 | 21.9 | 22.9 | 23.9 | 24.9 |

Underweight Normal Overweight Obesity

## 8. History of medication use

Certain medications also carry the risk of impairing fertility including anti-depressants, acne treatments, tranquilizers and narcotics. Additional medications known to reduce fertility include:[cvii]

- Agamet (cimetidine) for treatment of peptides and ulcers
- Dilantin (phenytoin)- medication used to treat epilepsy
- Folex (methotrexate)- drug that stops replication of cells, used for chemotherapy
- Axulfidine (sulfasalazine)- medication used to treat autoimmune conditions like Crohn's disease, ulcerative colitis, rheumatoid arthritis
- Corticosteroids- steroid hormones

- Chemotherapy drugs such as Cytoxan and Neosar (cyclophosphamide)
- Sulfasalazine- anti-inflammatory used for IBS or rheumatoid arthritis
- Androgens- can impact male reproductive function
- Testosterone- (spironolactone, Ketoconazole, cyproterone acetate)
- Androgenic antagonists (spironolactone, cyproterone acetate, flutamide, cimetidine)
- Ejaculatory and erectile function inhibitors
- Antihypertensive drugs (methyldopa, reserpine, β-blockers, clonidine)
- Antipsychotic or neuroleptic drugs (phenothiazine, butyrophenone, lithium)
- Antidepressive or antidepressant drugs (tricyclic antidepressants, monoamine oxidases inhibitors)
- Anticholinergic agents- drugs to inhibit involuntary parasympathetic nerve impulses
- Recreational drugs

## B. Testing

Oftentimes, testing begins with a physical exam before delving into technologies that allow us to take a much deeper look at what may be going on. For both the man and the woman, there are physical signs that help us to reach a diagnosis. Physically, I look at a woman's hair growth (body and head), breast discharge that can indicate elevated prolactin and luteal phase discharge, abnormal thyroid growth, skin and weight. For the man, it is important to have a thorough physical examination of the genetalia, even when there is no reported concern with fertility. A urologist will look closely for a normal penis, scrotum, testes, size, nodules and any sign of a variocole, a condition which impacts the temperature of the testes and production of sperm.

I like to use ultrasound in both men and women, because they can reveal more than we can see with our bare eyes. Even though some doctors feel it is controversial to use ultrasound if all it reveals is a small variocole (which may or may not impact fertility), I believe it is important as an explorative tool. Furthermore, for the woman, a pelvic vaginal ultrasound is much more accurate and not as uncomfortable as using your hands to examine the vagina and abdomen. Using the ultrasound allows us to confirm the shape of the uterus and the presence of fibroids that could affect blood flow and implantation. Seeing the ovarian size and determining whether or not there are follicles or small cysts in the ovaries helps to diagnose normal follicle reserves and cases of polycystic ovaries. Sometimes you can also identify endometrial cysts, indicating endometriosis or dilated, fluid-filled fallopian tubes (hydrosalpinx), resulting from a pelvic infection.

When further investigation is indicated, after the

pelvic exam and ultrasound, we move on to more in-depth tests to aid diagnosis, including some or all of the following:

A **laparoscopy** is a minimally invasive surgery that allows the surgeon to view the pelvic organs through a small incision in the belly button. The client is placed under general anesthesia and the abdomen is inflated with gases so a thin, long tube with a lighted camera can be gently guided into the abdomen. The camera allows the surgeon to view and captures images of the condition of the pelvic organs. The organs of major interest include the outside of the uterus, ovaries and fallopian tubes. A laparoscopy can diagnose endometriosis (abnormal growth of endometrial tissues), fibroids (non-cancerous growths in the uterus), cysts, adhesions (scar tissue), hydrosalpinx (fallopian tube with a build up of fluid), and infections, which may be causing infertility. During a laparoscopy, many of the issues detected can be fixed, improving your chances of conceiving. A laparoscopy is an out patient procedure that lasts 1-3 hours, plus 1-2 hours of recovery time. Clients can return to work within a week.

A **hysteroscopy** is a less invasive surgery that allows the surgeon to view the inside of the uterus. The client is placed under a light sedation to ensure comfort. The cervix is dilated, and a thin, long tube with a lighted camera is placed in the uterus. The surgeon can view the lining of the uterus, and look for adhesions (scar tissue), endometriosis (abnormal growth of endometrial tissues), fibroids (non-cancerous growths in the uterus), polyps (excess tissue growth), septum (tissue growth which divides the uterus), and infections. During a hysteroscopy many of the issues detected can be remedied, increasing your chances of conceiving. A hysteroscopy is an out patient procedure that typically lasts 30-45 minutes, plus 1–1.5 hours of recovery time. Clients can return to work within 1-2 days, depending upon how they are feeling.

**Laparoscopy with hysteroscopy** – Often, the surgeon will perform both procedures together to create a full diagnostic picture. Clients will be put under general anesthesia and can return to work within a week.

To reveal any blockages in the fallopian tubes, we use a **hysterosalingography** (HSG) test where radiographic contrast dye is inserted into the uterine cavity through the vagina. If the tubes are open, they will fill up, and the dye will overflow into the pelvic cavity. HSG's are extremely useful in determining the existence and location of a tubal blockage, an irregularly shaped uterus, and intrauterine adhesions that indicate Asherman's Syndrome.

A **hysterosonogram** also reveals any abnormalities in the uterus and ovaries. During this procedure, we insert a speculum into the vagina, followed by a tube that pumps a saline solution into the cervix to expand the uterus, using an ultrasound probe intra-vaginally to look for fibroids, causes of miscarriage, uterine lining abnormalities and growths.

**Additional Diagnostic Testing**

Beyond the physical examination, there are a number of tests that are helpful in the diagnostic phase:

**Semen and Sperm Analysis:** We always test the man's sperm regardless of whether or not they have fathered children in the past, and regardless of whether or not they have been tested in the past and received "normal" results. Because sperm samples can be affected by so many factors--including time of last ejaculation, medications, diabetes, and hypertension--I always repeat sperm testing two weeks after an abnormal test and request blood tests that will indicate hormonal imbalance, genetic conditions and long-term disease as influences in sperm health.

The process of semen collection involves having the man masturbate into a cup after 3 days of abstinence to observe sperm count, motility and morphology. After ½ an hour to 2 hours, we test the volume of semen present in an ejaculate sample. Once the semen has liquefied (approximately 30 minutes), we can measure the percentage of mobile sperm, the count and the morphology present in a single drop of semen through use of a microscope. With the human eye or computer models, we use a grid system to determine whether the sperm values are normal:[cviii]

| Volume | 1.5- 5.0 milliliters |
|---|---|
| Sperm | 20 million per milliliter |
| Motility | Over 60% |
| Morphology | Greater than 14% are normal shape (strict criteria) |

**Beyond Count, Motility and Morphology:** A rather new revelation is the presence of DNA fragmentation: a condition that makes sperm incapable of producing pregnancy, despite normal or abnormal count, motility and morphology measures. This finding may explain many cases previously diagnosed as unexplained and is best discovered through a test called the Sperm Chromatin Structure Assay (SCSA). In this test, a frozen sperm sample is sent to the laboratory where it is thawed and subjected to a stress, like low ph. An orange- colored dye is applied to thousands of sperm, which is then passed under a beam of light, revealing either green (normal sperm) or orange (damaged DNA sperm). A computer counts the percentage of normal versus damaged sperm and assigns a DNA fragmentation index (DFI). Through analysis studies have revealed that men with damage less than 15% are likely to conceive where men with damage above 30% are not, and are more likely to have other abnormalities that cannot be measured.[cix] The causes of DNA fragmentation are assumed to be the same causes for other sperm decline, including toxin exposure, heat, variocole, infection, age, cancer, radiation and anything else that increases the prevalence of free radicals.

### Functional Tests

**Postcoital testing (PCT)** evaluates the relationship between the sperm and the cervical mucous two to eight hours after intercourse to ensure there is no immune reaction, such as sperm antibodies, and to evaluate sperm presence and motility in the case where the male partner does not want to be tested. Antibodies in the sperm can also be detected by collecting a sperm sample or by testing a woman's blood for the presence of an allergic reaction. The presence of antibodies can indicate **immunologic infertility.**

**Sperm penetration tests** measure whether the sperm is able to make it through the cervical mucus and fallopian tubes to meet and fertilize the egg. A mucus penetration test looks at the sperm's ability to persevere through the cervical mucous, whereas a penetration assay test combines sperm with hamsters' eggs in a laboratory to come up with a sperm capacitation index: the number of sperm that were able to penetrate the eggs.

**Hypo-osmotic swelling (HOS)** evaluates the integrity of male sperm by exposing sperm to hypo-osmotic solution to swell sperm tails. A low percentage of swelling has been correlated with reduced sperm motility and ability to fertilize an egg.[cx] HOS tests have been found to help determine which men will have trouble impregnating their partners through natural conception and IUI, and have higher rates of miscarriage due to damage in spermatozoan structure.[cxi]

## Blood Tests

Taking blood tests from both partners is a reliable way to test hormone levels, which may indicate endocrine imbalance as a factor in infertility. Blood tests may also reveal blood sugar imbalances, digestive disorders, genetic mutations and sub optimal nutrient levels that may be impacting your fertility. The following is a comprehensive list of tests with a brief description of what we are looking for:

## Hormone Panel

**Follicle Stimulating Hormone (FSH)** is tested on day 3 and is used as an indication of ovarian reserve (normal values 3-20mlU/ml). As women move towards menopause, FSH results are higher, indicating a lowering ability to stimulate the ovaries to produce follicles and release eggs. In men, FSH tests can help to diagnose low sperm count if levels are above 1-18 mIU/ml. This test will also be done when you have a baseline ultrasound for injectable gonadotropins for Intra-uterine insemination or In-vitro fertilization.

**Estradiol** is the form of estrogen tested in conjunction with FSH on day 3 and in elevated numbers (above 25-75 pg/ml.) It can indicate issues with ovulation and lowered ovarian reserve. Elevated estradiol can also suppress FSH levels, making that test inaccurate. In women, **low estrogen levels** may be indicated by hot flashes, headaches, night sweats and vaginal dryness, and interfere with the normal communications between the HPO axis and inhibit ovulation. In men, lower levels of estradiol were found (less than 10-60 pg/mL) in azoospermic or oligozoospermic infertility clients when compared with a group of proven fertile men.[cxii] Also indicated were lower levels of testosterone. This test will be done routinely when you have a baseline ultrasound for injectable gonadotropins for Intra-uterine insemination or In-vitro Fertilization. Estradiol levels will also be monitored approximately every 2 days during the stimulation stage of your cycle. **Thyroid (TSH)** is also taken on day three and either too much (hyperthyroidism > .4-4 uIU/ml) or too little (hypothyroidism= <.4-4 uIU/ml) can disturb your cycles creating infertility, and even recurrent miscarriage. Hypothyroid in particular can wreak havoc as the HPO axis can sense an underactive thyroid, and releases excess of other hormones to induce it to regulate, including prolactin. Elevated prolactin suppresses LH and FSH and their stimulation of the ovaries, interfering with ovulation. Excess thyroid can block estrogen, causing the uterine lining to be inadequate in thickness.

**A Progestin Challenge** is sometimes used to determine why there is a lack of ovulation (anovulation) or lack of period (ammenorhea). In this test, a pill form of progesterone is given anywhere from one to five days to see if menstruation is triggered. If bleeding does not occur, it means that a healthy dose of estrogen is being produced; if bleeding does occur, a woman is not making enough estrogen.

**Luteinizing Hormone** in women helps to regulate ovulation and shed empty follicles into corpus luteum. LH is required to produce ovulation and thus low levels of LH (day 3= < 7 mIU/ml, surge day= > 20 mIU/ml) in the blood stream can help to diagnose annovulation, ovarian failure, PCOS, pituitary disorders (low levels) and chromosomal abnormalities (high levels). LH urination test kits may also be used at home to indicate whether ovulation has occurred. In men, LH levels (below 2-18 mIU/ml) govern the production and creation of testosterone in the testes.

**Serum Progesterone** is an important indicator of a women's ability to carry a pregnancy to term. Progesterone levels rise in the blood after ovulation and peak from day 5-9 (ideally at 10ng/mL) declining a couple days prior to menstruation. If not enough progesterone is being produced the uterine lining will not be plush to preserve a growing fetus and often results in miscarriage. One study revealed that of fifty women who had been experiencing infertility for over a year and a half and were given progesterone cream, seventy percent conceived within six months.[cxiii] In men, progesterone (normal level= 15ng/mL to 100 ng/mL) is the building block for cortisol, testosterone and estrogen, among other hormones. When depleted, it can cause hormonal imbalance, including estrogen dominance. Progesterone is also recommended to reduce prostate enlargement and may help with a low libido. This test is performed when you have a baseline ultrasound for injectable gonadotropins for Intra-uterine insemination or In vitro Fertilization. It can also be performed during the midpoint of a client's cycle to help determine if the client is pre-ovulatory or post-ovulatory.

**Prolactin** is the hormone most often associated with breast milk production. High levels of prolactin (more than 20 ng/ml) reduce gonatropins and inhibit ovulation. When a woman is not pregnant, high levels of prolactin can indicate hypothyroidism or pituitary adenomas. Elevated prolactin can also be caused by some medications, including anti-psychotics. Symptoms include visual issues, headaches and breast discharge. In men, high levels of prolactin (more than 15ng/mL) can cause decreased testosterone and irregularities in sperm. Symptoms include impotence, low libido, low sperm count and hypogonadism (inability of testicles to produce proper amounts of sperm).

**Testosterone deficiency** (below 270-1100 ng/dl) in men is called hypogonadism, a main cause of infertility. Low testosterone can lower sperm count, cause low libido and erectile dysfunction, while also leading to enhanced feminine characteristics including breasts, less muscle mass, reduced facial and body hair resulting from estrogen dominance. Low testosterone combined with low FSH and LH can also indicate hypogonadotropic hypogonadism. Women secrete a small amount of testosterone from the adrenal glands and ovaries (normal values 6-86 ng/dl). High amounts of androgens in the form of testosterone in women often bring an increase in male sex characteristics such as lowered voice, decreased breast size, facial hair. It is most common in disorders like PCOS and also exists in less common conditions like Acromegaly, Adrenal neoplasm disorders, Conn's Syndrome, Cushings, Dwarfism, Gigantism, Multiple endocrine neoplasm 1 and 2, an androgen-producing adrenal or ovarian tumor, congenital adrenal hyperplasia and thyroid disorders.

**hCG (Human Chorionic Gonadotropin):** This test will be done when you have a baseline ultrasound for injectable gonadotropins for Intra-uterine insemination (IUI) or In-vitro Fertilization (IVF). It will also be ordered after an IUI or IVF cycle to assess whether pregnancy was achieved. Once pregnancy has been established, hCG levels might be monitored the first 2-3 weeks depending on the levels of hormone present.

## Additional Testing

**Iron levels** give us an indication of whether or not a woman is anemic, (normal levels 30-200). In a 2006 study, women who took iron supplementation were less likely to experience ovulatory infertility and it was shown that a lack of iron could be a root cause of infertility.[cxiv] Some prenatal supplements do not include iron, because some people are not deficient, and at heightened levels it can be toxic. Take your iron with meals, as it requires hydrochloric acid to be functional.

**Digestive disturbances** including inflammatory bowel disease (Crohn's and ulcerative colitis) as well as Celiac's Disease, the inability to tolerate gluten in foods, are associated with infertility in both men and women. A simple blood test can indicate whether you are in fact gluten intolerant, in which case dietary adjustments can help to ensure nutrients are being properly absorbed into your body.

**Glucose levels:** By studying blood sugar levels we can ascertain the effects of insulin resistance or metabolic syndrome, a precursor to diabetes. Recent studies have shown that women with PCOS commonly have metabolic syndrome, which increases levels of male hormones, causing infertility.

## Genetic Testing

" It was once thought that each of us arrived into adulthood already formed, our DNA locked into place, but this is not true. Studies show that our environment continues to encode the epigenomes and therefore alter our DNA. Not only that, the evidence shows that decisions encoded in the epigenomes can be passed down from one generation to the next- perhaps for several generations. What affected your grandmother might still be affecting you. What you do will be passed down to your great grandchildren."[cxv] —The Subtle Body Encyclopedia

### Preimplantation Genetic Diagnosis (PGD)

Preimplantation Genetic Diagnosis is an advanced technique, which allows individual embryos to be analyzed on a genetic level. This screening method is accurate approximately 90% of the time. This process is performed in conjunction with IVF, and involves the removal, fixation and analysis of a cell(s) from developing embryos. Depending on the genetic condition being screened for, examination of these cells may be performed by fluorescent in situ hybridization (FISH) or polymerase chain reaction (PCR). Genetic markers for certain diseases, such as cystic fibrosis, are tested utilizing PCR. Chromosomal abnormalities may be identified through FISH analysis.

At CNY Fertility Center, embryo biopsy is performed on the cleavage stage embryo on Day 3. (Egg retrieval and fertilization is designated Day 0). At this time, the embryologist will make a small opening in the zona pellucida (shell) of the egg, and remove one blastomere (cell) of the embryo using a small pipette. The embryos are placed back in the incubator to continue to grow. The cell will be fixed on a slide or placed in a tube according to the analysis, which is to be performed. The material to be tested is sent to the laboratory performing the analysis. Results are generally produced in 24-48 hours, so that an embryo transfer may be performed on Day 5.

PGD is recommended for clients who are affected by or carriers of a genetic anomaly in an attempt to drastically reduce the probability of passing the condition to their offspring. PGD may also be indicated in clients of advanced maternal age or with a history of recurrent pregnancy loss. PGD offers a means for family balancing, as the gender of the embryo may be determined through chromosomal analysis. PGD may reduce the chance of pregnancy by about 10%.

Genetic testing may be helpful in diagnosing a cause of either male infertility or female infertility. Through a series of tests including a chromosome analysis, your genes are studied to see if there are any mutations, which may be preventing you from conceiving. If genetic abnormalities are found, genetic counseling is highly recommended.

During a chromosome analysis a picture of your genes, also called a karotype, is taken to look for the following:

*For women:*

Changes in chromosome structure
Changes in chromosome numbers
Alterations in Fragile X region of the X chromosome

*For men:*

Changes in chromosome structure
Changes in chromosome numbers
Y deletion: missing regions of the Y chromosome
Alterations in the cystic fibrosis gene

Chromosome analysis may also reveal some of the

common causes of infertility in men and women as well as provide an explanation in the case of recurrent pregnancy loss.

**Some of the most common genetic conditions that impact fertility include are:**

**Klinefelter Syndrome** (47,XXY) affects men who are born with an extra X chromosome (instead of XY, they have XXY or XXXY or XXXXY). The condition causes female characteristic including enlarged breasts, small testes, lack of body hair and in some cases mild retardation. Klinefelter syndrome is the genetic cause of azoospermia (lack of sperm). Though some men with Klinefelter syndrome have fathered children from sperm found in their epidermis through use of intracyoplasmic sperm injection (ICSI) and in vitro fertilization, most often men use donor sperm or adopt.

**Turner Syndrome** (45, X) affects the development of a woman's ovaries through a missing X chromosome. In this case a woman generally has 45 pairs of chromosomes as opposed to the normal 46. Physical characteristics include being short, having a webbed neck and often times the condition is diagnosed before issues of infertility arise. Turner Syndrome can manifest in a few different ways, from two identical cell lines with one X chromosome missing, to part of the genetic material missing off the one X chromosome.

Women with Turner Syndrome may opt to move forward with an egg donor, or depending on their pathology, may be candidates for IVF.

**Translocations** are found in 2-5% of couples who experience recurrent miscarriages. Passed down from either the mother or the father, a re-arrangement of chromosomes occurs during cell division, impacting the genetic material and outcome. In a balanced translocation, no genetic material is lost or gained, but it is now in the wrong location. In the case of familial translocation, the mother and father may have no symptoms whatsoever, and only genetic testing can reveal the lineage. Sometimes, in the case of de nova translocation, the genetic rearrangement occurs for the first time during conception, due to the way the chromosomes are wrapping around each other in cell division. A couple who is affected by translocations may choose to continue with natural conception, use donor sperm or eggs or try IVF with preimplantation genetic diagnosis (PGD) where the chromosomes of the human embryo are carefully monitored for genetic defects prior to implantation.

**Fragile X Syndrome**: Women who carry a permutation of Fragile X have a 14-16% greater risk of developing Premature Ovarian Failure, which impacts 1% of the population. Women who carry a permutation of Fragile X are more likely to have babies that develop a full mutation of Fragile

X syndrome, so genetic counseling is strongly advised in this case. Women impacted by Fragile X may experience lower success rates with reproductive treatments and response to medications. Options include conceiving earlier in life to mitigate effects of POF, utilizing PGD with IVF if you determine prenatal diagnosis is important to you prior to birth, or using donor eggs.

**Cystic Fibrosis** is believed to affect 30,000 children and adults in the US alone with over 10 million unaffected carries. Cystic Fibrosis impacts the digestive system and respiratory tracts, causing a sticky mucous to form making it difficult to breathe, thereby increasing lung infections and making it more difficult for the pancreas to break down food and absorb nutrients. Whether men have the symptoms of CF or not, geneticists look for the 32 common mutations related to the cystic fibrosis gene, which is a cause of CBAVD, or congenital bilateral absence of the vas deferens, where the tube which releases the sperm to the testes is underdeveloped as though the man has had a vasectomy, resulting in infertility. Women are not regularly screened for the gene mutations, though they may experience complications in fertility or pregnancy as a result of worsening CF symptoms. Men may proceed with assisted reproductive technology through in vitro fertilization or ICSI.

**Y Deletion** is the second leading genetic cause of male infertility besides Klinefelter syndrome. In Y deletion, a microscopic part of the genetic material in the Y chromosome passed from the father to the son is missing, resulting in azoospermic factor or low sperm count. Microdeletion is detected through specialized, advanced genetic techniques like polymerase chain reaction (PCR) which look closely at the "AZF" region of the Y chromosome to determine which areas and how much are missing. In men with no sperm, ART may be used to retrieve sperm from the epidermis for In Vitro Fertilization. Many men opt to use donor sperm when it cannot be retrieved or when they have decided on their own or through genetic counseling that they do not want to pass the Y chromosome to their offspring in the case that it is a son. In the case where a couple uses their own sperm, they may opt to pre-select a female embryo as to not pass on the Y deletion.

**Histocompatibility** occurs when the couple has an exact or close to exact match of genes referred to as the "major histocompatibility complex." This set of genes exists in the tissues and is viewed as antigens to the body for which it makes antibodies.

**Mullerian agenesis** is an inborn abnormality in which no vagina or uterus develops in the female embryo. These women may choose to use IVF alongside with a surrogate mother to have their fertilized egg implanted.

**Kallman Syndrome** is a genetic disorder implicated in 20% of Idiopathic hypogonadotropic hypogonadism cases, where abnormalities in the hypothamulus result in the underproduction of FSH and LH resulting in underdeveloped ovaries and infertility.

**Congenital adrenal dysplasia (CAH)**[cxvi] defines a category of genetic disorders where the adrenal hormones aren't produced in proper amounts or at all. Each year, one in 14,000 babies is born with CAH, which impacts the adrenal glands' ability to help in the formation of the endocrine system. Normally, the adrenal hormones including adrenaline, aldosterone, cortisol and androgens are converted from cholesterol through one of the enzymes that is deficient in those affected by CAH. The disorders are named after the specific hormone that is deficient:

- 21-hydroxylase deficiency (most common-blocks cortisol)
- 11-beta-hydroxylase
- 3-beta-hydroxysteroid dehydrogenase
- 17-alpha-hydroxylase (very rare)

Babies born with CAH may find:

- Production of cortisol is blocked, which limits the body's ability to deal with stress, maintain steady blood sugar levels, support

the immune system and steady blood sugars
- Overproduction of androgens (male sex charactertics)
- An inability to produce the sodium-regulating hormone, aldosterone resulting in "salt losers" which affects blood sugar and blood pressure.

Classic cases of CAH are described as salt losers or "non-salt losers." Both are marked by low cortisol resulting in excess male sex characteristics or androgens.

**"Salt losers" -** 8 out of 10 CAH cases are salt losers, with insufficient aldosterone, meaning the kidneys excrete too much salt, which dries up the water and fluids in the body, impacting blood volume and pressure. Salt losers suffer from dehydration, vomiting, nausea and adrenal crisis, which occurs when potassium levels rise due to plummeting salt, creating a potentially life threatening situation.

**"Non salt losers" -** The other 2 out of 10 are considered non salt losers or "virilising CAH," and though they have sufficient levels of aldosterone, they are lacking cortisol and overly abundant in androgens. The masculinising effect is often recognized in baby girls at birth who experience enlarged clitoris and a partial fusion in the lips of labia. Boys may go through puberty at the early age of 2 or 3 years old, developing penis and pubic hair.

**Non-Classical "late onset" -** Usually involves a milder gene mutation where the symptoms often times develop later in life, though not always. Signs and symptoms include early pubic hair growth, acne, body odor, facial hair, irregular menstrual cycle and infertility. Oftentimes cortisone medications are used to correct androgen excess.

**CAH and women -** In particular, CAH can cause structural problems for women who are often born with ambiguous male/female genitals because of the androgen excess. Surgery is used to separate the labia and trim the clitoris so that sexual intercourse is possible.

**Cushing's Syndrome**[cxvii] involves a group of hormone disorders characterized by an over-production of cortisol circulating through the body. Cortisol is produced by the adrenals and regulated by adrenocorticotropin (ACTH), which is secreted by the pituitary gland when cortisol levels drop too low. When cortisol levels are too high, the body will stop making ACTH in an attempt to slow cortisol production. This is sometimes caused by glucocorticoid hormone used to treat conditions like lupus, asthma and rheumatoid arthritis or may otherwise be caused by tumors in the pituitary and adrenal glands.

Symptoms of Cushing's include irregular menstrual cycles, ammenorrhea, frequent urination, high white blood cell count, susceptibility to pneumonia, weakened muscles, osteoporosis, round "moon shaped" faces, fat deposits between the shoulder blades, easy bruising, water retention, headaches, mood swings, abnormal hair growth as in PCOS and high blood pressure. Maintaining "normal" cortisol levels is important for the following functions:

- Moderate stress
- Balance blood sugar levels
- Decrease inflammation
- Regulate blood pressure
- Support immunity

Treatments options include surgically removing the tumor and depending on the location of the tumor hormone therapy, chemotherapy, immunotherapy and radiation therapy may be adjunct treatments. In some cases, glucocorticoid hormone therapy reverses the effects of Cushing's Syndrome, but the symptoms return as soon as the drugs are stopped.[cxviii]

**CNY Fertility's Checklist for Basic Fertility Testing**

Preconception Panel:

When this is drawn you can expect 7 tubes of blood to be taken. While this sounds like a large amount, it is about 50 ml or less.

- Estradiol
- Progesterone
- Human Chorionic Gonadatropin
- Thyroid Stimulating Hormone
- Prolactin
- Qualitative Rubella IgG
- Follicle Stimulating Hormone
- CBC (complete blood count) with a differential
- ABO/RH and antibody screen
- RPR
- Hepatitis B Surface Antigen
- Varicella Zoster IgG
- Cystic Fibrosis
- Thyroid Stimulating Hormone
- Prolactin
- Rubella IgG
- HIV

Additional Tests Recommended with Recurrent Pregnancy Loss:

- Karyotype testing
- Lupus Anti-Coagulant
- Anti-Nuclear Antibody

Prenatal Panel (to be ordered once pregnancy is achieved): Note: Not all of these tests need to be repeated if they have been done previously.

- CBC with a differential

- ABO/RH and antibody screen
- RPR,
- Hepatitis B
- Surface Antigen
- Varicella Zoster IgG
- Cystic Fibrosis
- Thyroid Stimulating Hormone
- Rubella IgG
- HIV

## C. Treatments

After thoroughly testing both partners and identifying potential factors contributing to a couple's infertility, treatment options will be recommended based on their individual needs. Not all couples and individuals need the most advanced treatments as the first course of action. Conversely, couples and individuals with identifiable factors may experience no benefits from the simpler protocols.

**Clomid citrate** is commonly the first medication that is prescribed for clients who are unable to ovulate empirically with unspecified infertility in combination with insemination. Women who have normal fallopian tubes, regular 28-day cycles and partners with a normal sperm count, but are still experiencing infertility, are termed as having 'unspecified' infertility.

**FSH & LH -** The pituitary gland regulates the amount of FSH (follicle stimulating hormone) and LH (luteinizing hormone) in the system. These two hormones play a key role in ovulation. The levels of these hormones determine when and how many eggs are developed and released. LH is responsible for the further maturation and release of the egg(s).

**Increasing FSH & LH -** Clomid citrate is an anti-estrogen medication. This means that it tricks the pituitary gland into thinking that the levels of estrogen in the body are low, causing the pituitary gland to secrete additional FSH and LH. This increase of FSH and LH stimulates the development of the follicles that contain the egg(s). Clomid citrate is taken as a pill, and generally is prescribed as one (50mg) pill each day for 5 days in the beginning of the menstrual cycle (days 3-7). A mature follicle is usually found about 7 days after the last Clomid pill is taken.

**Monitoring Effectiveness -** If ovulation does not occur, the medication can be changed to reflect the client's needs. Ultrasound is the best way to determine the number and the maturity of the follicles. To establish if ovulation has occurred, ovulation predictor kits may be used. They determine if there has been a surge of LH mid-cycle, indicating ovulation has occurred. Ovulation occurs about 24-28 hours after the detection of the

LH surge in the urine. Once ovulation has occurred, natural or artificial insemination is done in an attempt to fertilize the egg(s) that have been produced.

Injectable medications are used for IVF or IUI cycles. One of the main processes in an IVF or IUI treatment cycle is the controlled stimulation of the ovaries, to produce eggs. The medications used in ovulation induction are called gonadotropins. Brand names include Follistim, Gonal-F, Menopur, Bravelle, and Repronex. Gonadotropins are primarily used to treat two types of women:

- Those who do not ovulate, ovulate irregularly, or have failed to conceive using Clomiphene citrate (Clomid).
- Women who ovulate on their own, but may need help in producing multiple eggs, and whose bodies would benefit from the enhanced hormonal environment.

**How Do They Work?**

Gonadotropins are natural hormones that trigger the ovaries to make eggs. They are generally safe to use, but do require experience and careful monitoring. In a natural menstrual cycle without any medications, a woman produces one or two follicles, which are fluid filled sacs that contain an egg. The secretion of two hormones from the pituitary gland influences the growth of the eggs and their release from the follicles: Follicle Stimulating Hormone (FSH); and Luteinizing Hormone (LH), both known as gonadotropins.

When a woman becomes menopausal, her pituitary gland secretes large amounts of these hormones in an attempt to stimulate the ovaries, which no longer function. Gonadotropins (other than Follistim and Gonal F) are manufactured by extracting FSH and LH from the urine of post-menopausal women. Menopur contains both FSH and LH, while Bravelle contains only FSH.

For a woman going through infertility treatments, these extracts must be injected and cannot be taken orally, because the stomach would digest them. Recently, gonadotropins (Gonal-F, Follistim) have been manufactured in the laboratory using recombinant technology, which allows a pure form of FSH to be produced. This is not a human tissue or urinary by-product; it is a recombinant FSH. Since it is more pure, it may be self-injected, using a small needle just under the skin.

Although the gonadotropin medication regimen may seem complicated and perhaps even confusing, it is a fairly easy process once you understand the steps, methods and effects.

**Injection Technique -** Several days before the first treatment cycle, you and your partner need to learn the proper technique for giving intramuscular and subcutaneous injections. You can borrow a VHS videotape demonstrating the injection technique from our office and you can also visit our website here http://cnyfertility.com/resources/injection-lessons/ to watch one of our nurses demonstrate the procedure. It is not difficult to learn, and can be mastered quickly. Our Nurse Coordinator can supervise your first injection and answer any questions.

**Baseline Ultrasound -** Gonadotropin injections are usually started about two to three days after you begin menstruating. On the first day of your period, you need to call our office to schedule a baseline ultrasound to detect any preexisting ovarian cysts. Ovarian cysts are very common, are often cyclical and usually resolve on their own. However, if a cyst is found, your treatment cycle may be altered or delayed. A vaginal probe is used for the ultrasound and is harmless to you and your developing eggs.

**Injections for Egg Development -** After the baseline ultrasound, you will be instructed when to begin your injections. Each woman's protocol, start date, dosage and length of treatment are unique and individual to her. Typically, you will be on the injections for three to five days before coming back into our office for your next ultrasound to evaluate follicular response. You may also have a blood test to measure the hormone estradiol, which is secreted by the growing follicles. The ultrasound/blood test is important not only to measure your progress, but also to monitor your ovaries for any abnormalities due to hyperstimulation. At the time of this ultrasound, you will be given instructions regarding injection dosage for that evening, the next day and schedule a time for your next ultrasound and blood test.

**Egg Release -** The follicles (the fluid filled sacs containing the eggs) are visualized and measured by ultrasound. Depending on the follicle growth and estradiol levels, variable doses of gonadotropins (FSH) are given for an additional three to seven days. When the ultrasound and blood tests indicate that the follicles are mature and ready to release the eggs, a single injection of human Chorionic Gonadotropin (hCG; brand names are Pregnyl or Profasi though generic is suitable) or a recombinant form known as Ovidrel, is given to induce ovulation, the release of the eggs. hCG is a natural hormone produced by the placenta and is similar to the LH hormone released monthly by the pituitary gland. Egg retrieval is usually thirty-six hours after this hCG injection. Intercourse should be avoided during this period.

**Progesterone Supplements -** After the eggs are inseminated, many clients receive progesterone in the form of injections, vaginal suppositories, vaginal cream or oral pills. Progesterone helps develop the lining of the uterus to allow the embryos to implant. If you are on progesterone, your menstrual cycle may be delayed even if you do not become pregnant. If your period is more than two to three days late, you should schedule a blood pregnancy test before stopping any progesterone supplementation.

IUI is used to treat infertility due to mild to moderate-low sperm count, abnormal sperm or marginal motility, poor cervical mucus, anti-sperm antibodies and unexplained infertility. IUI is the process by which prepared sperm is placed within the uterus around the time of ovulation. The pregnancy rate for IUI is about 3-6% per treatment cycle, but this success rate is dependent on the type and severity of the infertility problem. However, stimulating the ovaries to develop multiple eggs increases pregnancy rates to 9-20%.

**How is the IUI performed?**

An IUI is an office procedure. First, sperm is collected by masturbating into a clean cup. This can be done at home if it's within 30 minutes of the doctor's office, otherwise, it should be done at the office. The sperm is then prepared by washing it, a procedure that concentrates the most motile sperm into a small volume. There are three steps involved in washing the sperm:

- Removal of the seminal fluid, which contains proteins and hormones that can

cause painful uterine contractions and allergic reactions in the woman
- Isolation of the sperm that are most motile and most fertile
- Concentration of the sperm into a small volume comparable to the volume of the uterine cavity.

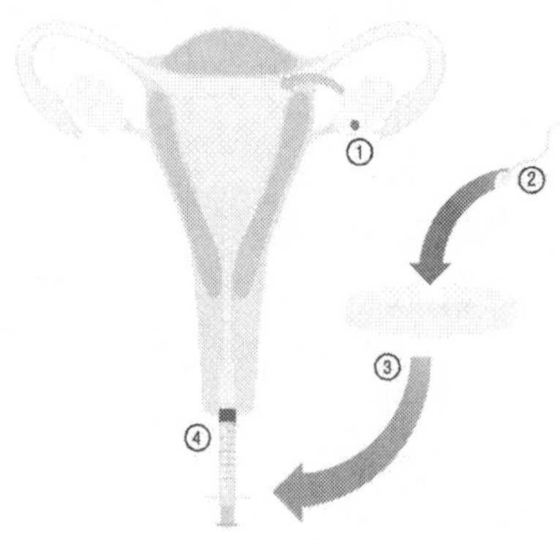


After the sperm is washed, it is placed into a small tube or catheter. This is passed through the cervix and into the uterine cavity. Then the sperm is ejected into the uterine cavity. Usually, this is a simple procedure that does not result in much discomfort. Some mild cramping can be expected. Rarely will an IUI be difficult and uncomfortable. However, in these situations, medications may be used to help ease any pain. The actual insemination only takes about 10 minutes. Afterward, the woman lies down for about 10 to 15 minutes and then can resume normal activity.

### When is it performed?

The IUI is performed as close to the day of ovulation as possible. Ovulation is usually determined by using a urinary LH ovulation test kit. These urinary ovulation test kits are available over-the-counter. Ovulation may also be artificially induced with an HCG injection. Insemination is usually performed the day after an HCG injection or positive LH test. The timing of ovulation is critical to increase the chances for pregnancy. Ovulation occurs about 38 to 42 hours after the LH is released into the blood stream. By taking daily urine tests before and around the time LH should be released, ovulation can be accurately predicted. It usually occurs 12 to 14 days before menstruation. If a woman has a regular 28-day cycle, ovulation should occur around day 14 (28-14=14). If a woman has a 30-day cycle, ovulation occurs around day 16 (30-14=16). Start testing about 4 days before anticipated ovulation. Sometimes, if a kit does not turn positive, you might think there is something wrong with it. If you have been testing for 5 days, and your kit has not shown positive, call the office for instructions. Be sure to carefully read the kit instructions and call the manufacturer with any questions regarding its use.

**What if my period is late?**

You can expect to menstruate about 2 weeks after the IUI if you are not pregnant. If you are using progesterone vaginal suppositories, your period may be late even though you may not be pregnant. If you are late and you suspect you are pregnant, call the office to schedule a pregnancy test. Generally, 3 to 6 cycles of IUI are performed before moving on to other fertility treatments.

# In Vitro Fertilization (IVF):

### Assisted Hatching (AH)

The assisted hatching technique consists of making a small opening in the zona pellucida (shell) that surrounds the embryo. Embryos must hatch from the zona pellucida prior to implanting in the uterus. Some evidence suggests that assisted hatching may make it easier for hatching to occur, and therefore may improve implantation rates. There is a small risk of damage to the embryo during the micromanipulation process or at the time of embryo transfer. Although some centers have reported a slight increase in identical twinning as a result of assisted hatching process, we have not observed this at our facility.

The methods currently used for assisted hatching are chemical (acid tyrode's), mechanical (partial zona dissection), and laser (heat). The laser technique is used at CNY Fertility Center. Prior to embryo transfer, the embryologist creates a small opening in the embryo's zona pellucida using a specially designed laser, which attaches to the microscope.

Assisted hatching is offered to all couples/individuals. In our center, we perform assisted hatching on nearly all of our cases as we feel it enhances implantation and pregnancy rates. It is most commonly recommended in conjunction with IVF for:

- Couples/Individuals undergoing IVF with the female partner's age 37 or older.
- Couples/individuals undergoing IVF that have had one or more previous failed IVF cycles.
- Couples/individuals undergoing IVF whose embryos have a thicker than usual zona pellucida.

**In Vitro Fertilization** (IVF) is an assisted reproductive technology (ART). IVF is an outpatient procedure done in our office. After a client is given gonadotropins to stimulate her ovaries, the oocytes (eggs) are aspirated, collected in a dish and inseminated.

The insemination may be conventional (adding sperm to the eggs allowing them to fertilize on their own) or via Intra Cytoplasmic Sperm Injection (ICSI) whereby one sperm is directly injected into an egg.

**The processes involved with IVF are:**

- Prevention of premature release of eggs from the ovaries
- Stimulate development of multiple eggs in the ovaries
- Removal of the eggs from the ovary
- Combining the eggs with sperm
- Embryo transfer
- Establishing pregnancy

**The In Vitro Fertilization process is as follows:**

- The eggs are harvested after medication therapy
- The eggs and sperm are either left together in an incubator for about 18 hours, (conventional IVF) or they are inseminated using ICSI, whereby one sperm is directly injected into the egg. They are then checked for fertilization and further development as embryos.
- The resulting embryos are placed in the uterus. Progesterone is also used to help develop the uterine lining and increase the chances of implantation.

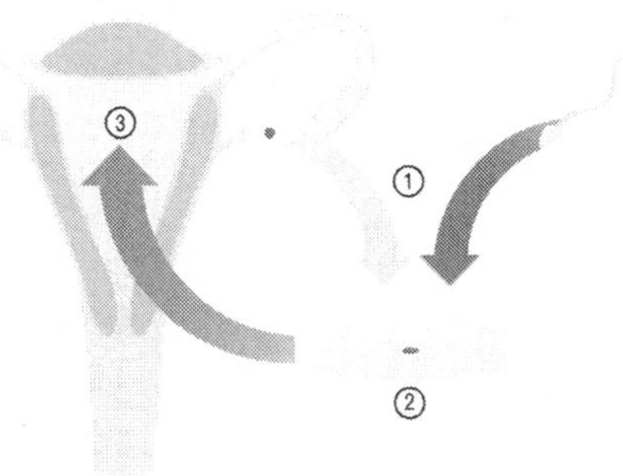


## Ovarian Stimulation

An IVF treatment cycle begins with the onset of a menstrual period. A week before the beginning of the next period, a medication called Lupron is administered. Lupron prevents premature release of eggs from the ovaries. Lupron is a very small daily subcutaneous injection given just under the skin. Any part of the body can be used for these shots and the woman or her partner can administer them. Lupron is given daily for about three to four weeks. Because estrogen levels are low, side effects may include fluid retention, headaches or hot flashes.

About a week after taking Lupron, your period will start. From this point on, Lupron will keep you hormonally "frozen" in that normal egg production is put on hold. A few days to a week from the start of your period, hMG injections will be taken along with the Lupron injections. Follistim, Gonal-F, and Bravelle are all collectively known as hMG, but you will only be injecting one of these medications. Lupron puts your ovaries on "hold," that is, prevents them from releasing the eggs before we are ready to collect them. At the same time, HMG stimulates development and maturation of multiple eggs in the ovaries. The objective of this medication protocol is to produce as many eggs as possible in a given cycle, and "tell" the ovaries to hold them until we are ready to collect them. On average, about 6 to 12 eggs develop.

CNY Fertility Center offers different protocols to ensure quantity and quality of eggs collected. An individualized treatment plan will be created for you at the time of your consultation/follow-up talk. Ovarian stimulation may begin 2-4 days after your period begins or one week before the start of your next period. The prevention of premature ovulation may be done using Lupron or other medications called antagonists known as Ganirelix or Cetrotide. Our physicians will determine which approach is best for you.

Before starting hMG injections, an ultrasound will be made of your ovaries to check that no cysts or large follicles exist. Injections in the form of Follistim, Gonal-F or Bravelle are shallow injections that are given just under the skin, usually in the abdomen or upper arm. Some side effects may occur with hMG injections, such as abdominal bloating, weight gain due to fluid retention and pelvic or abdominal discomfort or both. These are signs of ovarian hyperstimulation and usually do not require any treatment. It is rare for a woman to be hospitalized for severe symptoms.

You will be taking Lupron and hMG injections every day for about ten days. During these ten days, your progress will be monitored with ultrasound and possibly estradiol blood tests. Since the eggs are microscopic, they cannot be seen on ultrasound. However, we can see when the eggs are mature from the size of the ovarian follicles, or the fluid filled sacs within the ovaries that contain the eggs. These monitoring visits are brief and usually done in the morning

Once the eggs are almost mature, you will stop taking the Lupron and hMG. You will then take a single injection of hCG hormone. This medication triggers the final stages of egg maturation. The eggs are nonsurgically removed from the ovaries 36 hours after the hCG injection. You should not have intercourse during the time between the hCG injection and egg retrieval.

### Fertilization

### Oocyte (Egg) and Embryo Cryopreservation (Freezing)

Oocyte/embryo cryopreservation is a process where oocytes/embryos are immersed in a series of solutions, which dehydrate the cells and replace the water molecules with cryoprotectant, thereby protecting the integrity of the cells during the freezing process. The oocytes/embryos are loaded into specially designed straws, and placed into liquid nitrogen tanks for long-term storage. These frozen oocytes/embryos may be subsequently thawed and used for a future embryo transfer. Not all clients undergoing IVF will have embryos for freezing. Surplus embryos remaining after embryo transfer are evaluated, and if they have advanced appropriately developmentally, they may be frozen.

The two primary methods for freezing are slow freezing and vitrification. In the slow freeze method, the oocytes/embryos are incubated in a series of solutions designed to dehydrate the cells and replace water with cryoprotectant. The cryoprotected oocytes/embryos are loaded into straws, and placed in special freezers to slowly cool the embryos to a specified temperature over the course of 2-3 hours. The cooled straws are then stored in liquid nitrogen tanks.

Vitrification is a process whereby the water molecules are replaced with a higher concentration of cryoprotectant than in the slow freeze method as the oocytes/embryos are exposed to a series of solutions. The embryos are then plunged into liquid nitrogen, and transferred to liquid nitrogen tanks where they will be stored. This quick freezing reduces the chance for intracellular ice crystals to be formed, thus decreasing the degeneration of cells upon thawing for embryo transfer. Many studies have shown survival rates of vitrified embryos to be far higher than those of slow freeze embryos.

CNY Fertility Center now performs vitrification as the method for cryopreservation.

**Indications for cryopreservation include:**

Preserving surplus embryos following embryo transfer, which may be used in the future to achieve a pregnancy. By transferring frozen-thawed embryos into the uterus, it is possible to achieve 2 or more pregnancies in different years from a single egg retrieval.

Preserving fertility is valuable to clients who must undergo medical treatments such as chemotherapy for cancer treatment, which may affect fertility. By undergoing IVF with embryo freezing, the couple/individual may thaw and transfer cryopreserved embryos following successful treatment.

Oocyte (egg) freezing is currently considered investigational, as eggs are much more delicate than embryos when it comes to the freezing and thawing process. Although significant advances have been made in the technique, success rates are still lower than those from embryos. Oocyte freezing may be an option for long-term fertility preservation in situations where a female may require cancer therapy treatment, but currently does not have a partner and chooses not to fertilize her eggs with "donor" sperm. CNY Fertility center is currently performing oocyte cryopreservation on an investigational basis, as recommended by ASRM.

The number of eggs retrieved will depend upon your age and response to hMG. But on average, six to 12 eggs are developed. As soon as the eggs are identified under the microscope, they are placed in petri dishes that contain a culture medium. The prepared culture medium is a composition that so closely resembles your own body's fallopian tube secretion that the eggs, and subsequently the embryos, will develop in the petri dish just as they would in your body. The dishes are kept in an incubator at a constant temperature of 37°C, 100% humidity and 5% $CO_2$ concentration.

At the time of egg retrieval, the male partner will collect his sperm by masturbating into a clean cup. The semen is then washed and processed to remove the seminal fluid to get the highest quality sperm possible. It takes about four to six hours after retrieval for the eggs to finally mature to the point that they are ready for insemination. Traditionally, sperm has been added to each dish containing the eggs and letting nature take its course by fertilizing overnight. However, we are using ICSI even in normal cases to ensure that the best eggs are indeed fertilized. The fertilized eggs, now called embryos, continue to grow in the IVF laboratory. In three to five days, you will return for embryo transfer.

## ICSI

**Intracytoplasmic Sperm Injection (ICSI)**

ICSI is a method to fertilize eggs that was originally developed to circumvent male factor infertility. Currently, it is widely used in many IVF centers as the dominant fertilization technique even when semen parameters are normal. In vitro fertilization with ICSI is offered to all couples/individuals undergoing IVF- yet it is specifically recommended for:

- Couples with severe male factor infertility opting to use the male partner's sperm rather than donor sperm. Male factor infertility may be characterized by low sperm concentrations, low sperm motility, or very poor sperm morphology. Men who do not have sperm in their ejaculate often can undergo an office procedure under local anesthesia to remove sperm directly from the testes or epididymus.
- Couples who have previously undergone IVF cycles with no fertilization or a low rate of fertilization.
- Couples who have a low yield of eggs at egg

retrieval.
- Cycles in which PGS or PGD will be performed.

Intracytoplasmic sperm injection (ICSI) is a micromanipulation procedure developed to help couples with male factor infertility or previous low or failed fertilization. ICSI involves using a powerful microscope and an extremely small glass needle to physically inject a single sperm into the center of the woman's egg. After egg retrieval, the eggs that are most likely to be successful ICSI candidates are chosen. While holding the egg in place, the glass needle containing the single sperm is inserted into the egg and the sperm is injected directly into the cytoplasm, thereby fertilizing the egg.

Dr. Kiltz, along with the embryologist, will examine the embryos before transfer to determine the likelihood that any given embryo will implant. The quality of the embryos is very important. Several other factors may determine how many embryos will be transferred, such as your age, how many years you have been infertile and previous IVF cycles. Most couples with an average embryo quality usually select between two or three embryos to transfer. Generally, the pregnancy rate increases as more embryos are transferred, but so does the chance for multiple pregnancies. These issues will be discussed prior to your embryo transfer. The actual transfer is a brief procedure. The embryos are "loaded" into the tip of a catheter along with a very small amount of transfer medium. The catheter is then gently passed through the cervical canal and into the uterus. Usually, you never feel this. The embryos are slowly expelled near the top of the uterus. This transfer only takes a few seconds. No rest period is required after transfer and you can go back to your normal routine right away.

To help your body prepare itself for the embryos, you will be given daily progesterone to supplement your own. This additional progesterone starts the day of egg retrieval and continues for at least two weeks. Progesterone is a hormone that transforms the lining of the uterus to be an ideal receptor for the embryos.

After the embryo transfer, it's now up to nature. The front and back walls of the uterus gently squeeze the embryos and keep them in the uterine cavity. Your embryos cannot fall out, so there is no need to restrict physical or sexual activity. Even so, it might be wise to wait a few days before beginning any strenuous activity.

About two weeks after the eggs are retrieved, a blood test will be performed to determine if you are pregnant. This can be done at any lab of your choice. Your results should be available the same day. If the pregnancy test is positive, an ultrasound will be scheduled one week later to determine the implantation site. The heartbeat should be seen by four weeks after a positive pregnancy test. At this time, you will be given instructions regarding progesterone or other medication use.

Once a heartbeat is detected, there is a 90-95% probability that the pregnancy will continue to a live birth. There is only a 5-10% chance of miscarriage. IVF pregnancies are no higher a risk than natural pregnancies. After about 8 weeks into your pregnancy, you can return to your obstetrician for routine prenatal care.

If the pregnancy test comes back negative, you can stop the progesterone. Your period should start in a few days. You can begin another IVF cycle after one spontaneous menstrual cycle. Waiting will give your ovaries time to rest from the previous IVF treatment. There are several factors to consider before deciding on how many IVF cycles you may try before moving on to other treatments. These factors include your response, age, previous IVF cycles and the number of years you have been infertile. Just because you may not become pregnant after one, two or even three tries, does not automatically mean your chances of becoming pregnant are slim.

**A Typical IVF Calendar** *(based on 28-day menstrual cycle* please note: menstrual cycles vary in length)*

| SUNDAY | MONDAY | TUESDAY | WEDNESDAY | THURSDAY | FRIDAY | SATURDAY |
|---|---|---|---|---|---|---|
| 24 | 25 | 26 | 27 Lupron Injections | 28 | 29 | 30 |
| 31 | 1 Menses | 2 Baseline Ultrasound | 3 | 4 HMG Injections / Lupron Injections | 5 | 6 |
| 7 | 8 Ultrasound | 9 | 10 HMG Injections / Lupron Injections | 11 | 12 | 13 |
| 14 HCG | 15 | 16 Egg Retrieval | 17 | 18 Progesterone | 19 | 20 Embryo Transfer |
| 21 | 22 | 23 | 24 Progesterone | 25 | 26 | 27 |
| 28 | 29 | 30 Pregnancy Test | | | | |

## Additional options

### Donor Gametes

For couples and individuals who experience a lack of eggs or sperm, or whose eggs or sperm will not allow development into viable embryos, using donated eggs or sperm (or both in some cases) is a course of treatment worth consideration. Donors are usually anonymous, though not necessarily so – as in cases using family members or significant others.

### Oocytes (egg)

Egg donation is a viable option for women whose

ovaries no longer produce eggs or whose eggs cannot develop into viable embryos. It is also an option for those couples that wish to maintain a biological link, using the partner's sperm.

### Sperm

Sperm donation has been around for many years and has been socially acceptable for some time. Not only can a single woman, or women who do not have male partners, become pregnant using donated sperm, but males who have severe sperm abnormalities, or no sperm at all, or even potentially serious genetic traits he does not wish to pass on, can benefit. Donors are screened for STDs, heredity and genetic diseases and blood disorders. Donors can be found whom closely physically and mentally match the recipient. CNY Fertility Center does not maintain a donor sperm program, however, we can work with many different facilities and are happy to provide suggestions. If you choose your own facility, please confirm that they are licensed by the New York State Department of Health before purchasing or shipping donor sperm.

### Embryo

Embryo Donation is now another option available to our clients seeking to either create, or expand their families. Often when families undergo IVF treatments, they are left with remaining fertilized eggs (embryos). This can place the parents in a difficult position when they begin to discuss what to do with the remaining embryos. The previous options available have been to donate the remaining embryos to research, keep them frozen, or to dispose of them. We are now able to add a fourth option, Embryo Donation.

## Gestational Carrier

Gestational Carrier – client's eggs are fertilized with husband's sperm and then the resulting embryos are transferred into a third party's womb. The third party is the gestational carrier. The gestational carrier carries the pregnancy to term at which point she gives the baby to the genetic parents. The gestational carrier has no genetic link to the baby.

Using a gestational carrier has been a viable alternative for some time for women who may be able to produce eggs but not sustain a pregnancy. A woman who acts as a gestational carrier agrees to "provide a womb" for a couple who could not otherwise carry a baby through to birth. The intended mother's eggs are fertilized with the intended father's sperm through a regular IVF cycle. The resulting embryos are transferred to the gestational carrier, instead of the mother-to-be. Even frozen embryos can be used. If a woman cannot produce eggs, donor eggs are often used so there is no genetic link to the gestational carrier.

Using a gestational carrier is a much more involved process than even egg or sperm donation. In addition to the medical process each woman must to adhere to, a proper surrogacy arrangement is a complex legal contract involving responsibilities, and expenses. A lawyer who specializes in third-party reproductive law should handle this. Many times, friends or family members to great satisfaction and success carry out undocumented surrogacy "favors." But more often now, they are handled by agencies which specialize in surrogate arrangements. An agency will also provide proper psychological and medical screening that is critical to a successful surrogacy.

**Week Five: The right path for us**
**CNY Fertility client and blogger, April All Year**

In examining our approach to becoming parents, we knew that making an appointment with another fertility specialist was an absolute necessity. After unsuccessfully going through multiple IUI cycles, we were at a loss as to what the next best step was, but felt that consulting with CNY Fertility Center might offer a different perspective. Fortunately, our consultation with Dr. Kiltz was helpful and refreshing. During the hour-long visit, Dr. Kiltz did not focus solely on my cycle or my husband's sperm count. Instead, he focused on the fact that the possibility of our becoming parents was far more likely to happen than not and that our journey to parenthood had to involve what was best for us. We left the appointment feeling relieved for numerous reasons. First, we had a doctor who was listening to us and trying to thoroughly address our emotional and physical needs. Secondly, we left with a short-term plan, which included a series of different blood tests, continuing alternative treatments (acupuncture, massage, herbal remedies, etc.), initiating lifestyle changes (daily gratitude lists, meditating, yoga, etc.) and my undergoing a laparoscopy and hysteroscopy surgery.

I remember believing that surgery was the next best step. When there is no explanation for what is wrong with you, when your husband's "numbers" are fantastic, and you have failed many assisted cycles, all you want is an answer, other than a baby, that is! I felt that the surgery might offer some explanation. I knew it would be an invasive procedure, but that it only required small incisions (as long as there were no significant issues with my reproductive organs) and that this exploratory operation could be productive, depending on what the doctor found. The closer surgery date became, the more I knew that the doctor was going to find something that would provide an explanation for us. I do not know how I knew – call it intuition or call it coincidence, but I just knew. The first question I asked when I awoke from surgery was, "Did he find anything?" The nurse, who was phenomenal in terms of meeting my post-surgery needs, stated that I had a "spattering of things going on," and explained that the doctor removed endometriosis, scar tissue and a fibroid. I remember silently thanking God and smiling because I felt as if we now had several more puzzle pieces to lie into place.

I feel so much more hopeful now that we are working with a fertility center that meets our needs a bit more personally. My post-surgery follow-up visit was about 45 minutes, and we discussed the likelihood of achieving pregnancy and exactly what my chances of conception look like at this point (not too bad, I might add)! After discussing how my husband and I could continue to stay positive and spiritually "intact," we decided to simply relax until my two-month follow-up, at which point we would discuss our overall "fertility plan" with the doctor. As of today, our plan is in rough draft form, and developing our plan has been an emotional process, but I am determined to become a mother, and I have to be able to ask the tough questions and seek out the necessary answers.

Miracles and blessings,
*April all Year*

# Step 10: Empower with Information

As a doctor, one of the highest risks I see in giving a client a specific "diagnosis" is the tendency for it to become the center of their world. It's as though they have been given the key to unlock what is wrong and believe that if they spend all of their time gathering information on the problem, they will find the solution. Though it is our nature to seek out more knowledge, I have observed that seeking often becomes pathological and causes a level of stress that may do more harm than good.

In this age of Google, we have more information at our fingertips than we can possibly process. Most of you have no doubt experienced the panic that results when you Google a physical ailment and come up with a never ending list of consequences ranging in degree of severity from difficulty sleeping to death. And how do you sort through what is reliable and what is not? Does obsessive "Googling" bring you peace of mind or send you spiraling? Many of my clients experience "Google fear" resulting in paralyzing fear and worry that comes from focusing on what is wrong. We must remember that information is experiential evidence, and since each person is unique, it is important to be cautious of locking onto any absolutes in our discovery process. I always encourage clients to stay loose with the diagnosis and focus on the things that they can do to improve their fertility. Becoming overly connected to fear, worry and anxiety can block success. Focusing and holding tight to the problem never brings the solution. On a cellular level, fear contracts, and love expands. To liberate ourselves, we must find a different way of digesting information and diagnosis that leads us on a path to greater health and healing.

At CNY Fertility and CNY Healing Arts, our goal is to empower you with information to harmonize your mind, body and spirit. While some clinics operate on an antiquated patriarchal system, where your doctor hands you a prescription and you must either follow it to the letter or be released from their care, we at CNY believe you have the wisdom within you to choose your own healing journey. Our goal is to act as guides and provide you with all the options to support your fertility. Clients are encouraged to participate in the modalities that resonate with them and are welcome to change their mind along the way. So the question becomes how to present the material to you, and instill a confidence that propels you on a healing journey. That is my intention as your doctor: to see you achieve greater wellness and balance. Instead of limiting ourselves to a narrow definition, let us expand into the greater possibilities of healing by allowing information to empower us.

In this section, we will demystify the process of diagnosing infertility and share with you The Fertile

Secret protocols that use Western medicine alongside complementary medicine to treat your whole self and return your body to balance. Our Fertile Secret protocols are designed to support you through an integrative approach, not just from the Eastern or Western, and always to utilize the best path for the particular client. The best fertility protocol will consider a multitude of factors by addressing mind, body, and spirit, to prepare for pregnancy through the advances of Western medicine, Eastern healing therapies, diet and lifestyle, fertility massage, stress reduction and self reflection. As much as possible, I would encourage you to consider the myriad of ways we have to rebalance the body without getting "stuck" in the details of the diagnosis. None of these diagnoses mean that clients can't conceive naturally, but are rather factors that help to guide us on the treatment path. I have found it very important to focus your thoughts on exactly what you want: a healthy pregnancy with a baby in your arms. Positive intentions will make you more likely to be persistent in the plan described for you.

### The Fertile Secret's Holistic Approach to 10 Common Infertility Diagnoses

Advanced Maternal Age, Endometriosis, Fibroids, Recurrent Miscarriage, Luteal Phase Defect, Male Factor Infertility, PCOS, Premature Ovarian Failure, Structural Blockages, and Unexplained Infertility

## Advanced Maternal Age

### By definition…

Women who have been trying to conceive for over six months to a year without becoming pregnant and are 40 years of age or older are often given the diagnosis of "advanced maternal age" (sometimes this diagnosis is given as early as age 35). From the standpoint of Western medicine, a woman is born with all the eggs she will ever have and that the numbers decline from millions at birth to thousands when a woman is in her forties, making impregnation less likely. As one ages, physiologically, the blood flow decreases to the uterus and ovaries. At the same time, as a woman approaches menopause, the hormonal triggers from the HPO axis decline, lessening ovarian response and thereby declining egg quality and supply. As a result, women in their late 30's and early 40's are often introduced to more aggressive options, as outlined below to maximize opportunities for conception.

### Symptoms may include:

- High FSH levels
- Lack of follicles

## Western Medicine Testing and Treatments

**FSH Levels:** when FSH numbers begin to rise, we know that the body is working harder to stimulate the ovaries to release a follicle for implantation. The higher the FSH levels, the closer a women is to menopause where the process of ovulation will cease. Pre-menopausal FSH levels are generally below 13 mIU/ml. Several medications can help to stimulate ovulation and are often used in conjunction with IVF. In addition to serum FSH levels, day 3 estradiol, inhibin B and anti-Mullarian hormone can be helpful in diagnosing ovarian reserve.

**Antral Follicle Count (AFC):** Counting the follicles using an ultrasound is a reliable way to get an accurate idea of a woman's ovarian reserve. Generally there is not a significant fluctuation in the number of follicles from month to month so this test can give an accurate prognosis over time.[cxix] The ultrasound looks for follicles during days 2, 3, and 4, as they are beginning to grow. During this time, even a small amount of fluid will reveal follicles on the ultrasound as small as 2 mm and 5 mm. Antral follicles produce an echo that can be heard on the more highly sensitive transvaginal ultrasounds. Average numbers of follicles for the average mid 30's client are generally 5-10 follicles, while younger infertility clients may have up to 17. The antral follicle test is believed to be as accurate as biochemical methods of testing, according to a review of studies by Verkagen.[cxx]

## Hormonal Stimulation

1. Clomiphene citrate (clomid) induces ovulation through interaction with the pituitary gland. Clomid can help to increase the response of the ovaries despite elevated FSH levels, producing multiple eggs and therefore more opportunities for fertilization.
2. Follicle Stimulating Hormone (FSH) for injection, also known as Bravelle, Gonal-f, and Follistim in conjunction with Human Menopausal Gonadotropins (hMG,) also known as Menopur, are used to induce ovulation and are different than clomid, because it interacts directly on the ovaries.

## IVF or GIFT

Generally, this is the first course of treatment when a woman's fertility is waning. In combination with one of the above ovulation stimulators, a reproductive endocrinologist can retrieve multiple eggs from the ovaries, fertilize them with sperm, and re-insert into the uterus (IVF) or the fallopian tubes (GIFT). IVF results in twins 50% of the time, whereas GIFT has a lesser chance of multiples at 17%. GIFT is sometimes more appealing to a couple who wants to have a more natural approach, though it does involve a minor incision into the lower abdomen.

## Egg Donor

Nowadays, there is a surplus of frozen eggs, an estimated 400,000.[cxxi] For couples with have low ovarian reserve, donor eggs provide an opportunity to implant a healthy egg and carry a fetus through the gestational period. In a similar process to IVF, the egg is fertilized with the sperm and implanted into the uterus.

## A Chinese Medicine Perspective

The most common understanding of Oriental Medicine is that we are each born with a finite amount of "Jing" or life force (a signifier of our ovarian reserve) that we will treasure over our lifetime and exchange for life's activities. When a women appears to be entering menopause early, she often enters my office relaying experiences of hot flashes, a low libido, frequent urination, lack of blood flow during period, lack of cervical mucous, shorter cycles, an overall lack of fluids in the body, dry skin, thirst, along with the increase in FSH detected by her doctor. In order to treat elevated FSH and all signs of decreased communication in the HPO axis, we must restore a healthy flow between the meridians of the body primarily responsible for reproductive function: the penetrating, governing and conception meridians. By regulating these energetic systems and restoring a healthy balance of yin, we can often times restore a more youthful reproductive system and elongate a woman's fertility beyond the parameters of what Western medicine believes. Our goal is to reduce FSH by nourishing the blood and fluids of the body to regenerate the body's deepest reserves. The most common diagnosis of the western term "advanced maternal age" is a deficiency in kidney yin and blood, likely impacted by Liver Qi stagnation (the eastern equivalent of constriction and stress). In the treatment room, our favorite acupuncture points are Kidney 3 (to nourish yin), Liver 8 to nourish blood, and Zi Gong to bring more blood flow to the uterus and ovaries, urinary bladder 23 and 52 help to tonify and nourish the kidney, while back treatments with e-stim can help to bring more blood to the entire reproductive system.

Heightened FSH indicates a need to address Liver Qi stagnation through Liver 3, the herbal remedy xiang fu, which can be added to commonly used herbal treatments like six flavors, liu wei di wan tang or xiao yao san.

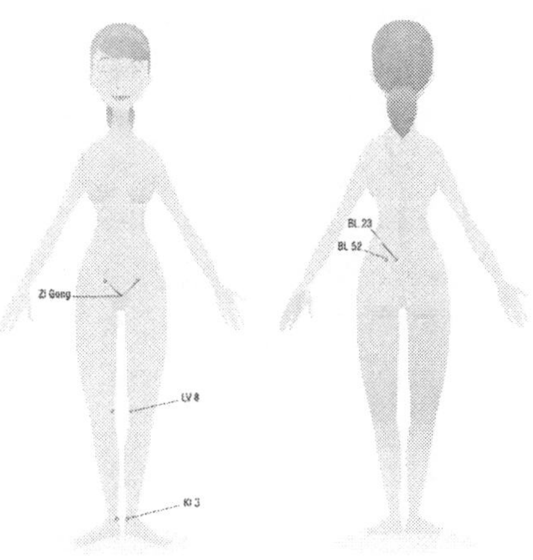


## Diet and Lifestyle Recommendations

A combination of exercise and nutrition can go a long way toward supporting restored reproductive function and defying the parameters of "advanced maternal age." Several studies have confirmed this belief showing that "dietary and endocrine manipulations can slow the pace of aging"[cxxii] along with evidence that a low-calorie diet fed to rodents slowed the disappearance of ovarian follicles.[cxxiii]

Above and beyond the general guidelines for eating for fertility, it is most important to build the yin and the blood.

**It is important to:**

- Eat yin-building foods like: adzuki beans,

black bean, bee pollen, blue-green algae, chlorella, clams, corn, gelatin, kelp, legumes, lycium, millet, mulberry, organ meats, oysters, parsley, pumpkin seed, raspberry, royal jelly, spirulina, string bean, tofu, walnuts, wheat germ, wheat grass, wild rice, yam.

- Restore and regenerate reproductive function, it is important to cut out any depleting lifestyle and dietary habits including stimulants like caffeine, alcohol, nicotine, unnecessary medications, street drugs along with toxins in the form of pesticides (always choose whole organic foods).
- Pay attention to how you are eating. Are you sitting down? Chewing slowly? How you eat is an important determinant of your stress levels, and relaxation is key for building up your fertility.
- Choose restful activities to build your energy reverses, exercising regularly but never overexerting. Exercise will help to send fresh oxygen and blood supply to your reproductive organs.

Supplementation for reducing elevated FSH and improving egg quality:

- High quality prenatal vitamin/mineral that includes 1,000 mcg folic acid
- CoQuinone– increases egg quality by

supporting mitochondrial function & energy production
- Wheat Grass – improves egg quality by lowering FSH levels
- Royal Jelly – improves egg quality by adding essential nutrients to the cells
- Fish oil – decrease inflammation, calms reactivity, increase uterine lining quality, overall support for hormonal balance, moderates NK cell activity
- DHEA- supports ovarian response (food source: extract of wild yams)
- L-arginine- increases blood flow to the uterus and ovaries (do not take if prone to herpes virus. Food sources: brown rice, chocolate, coconut, nut products, oatmeal, raisins, seeds)

**Massage Recommendations**

The Arvigo technique of Maya Abdominal Massage (ATMAM) can help to restore blood flow to the uterus and ovaries, thereby improving egg quality. If a couple chooses to proceed with a donor cycle, ATMAM can also help to thicken the uterine lining, making it more receptive to implantation. By increasing circulation, liver Qi stagnation is reduced, and the reproductive organs receive more nourishment. The process of working on the belly can be deeply relaxing and also help to connect the uterus and ovaries and gain a level of acceptance about the transformations occurring within the body.

**Ovarian Massage**

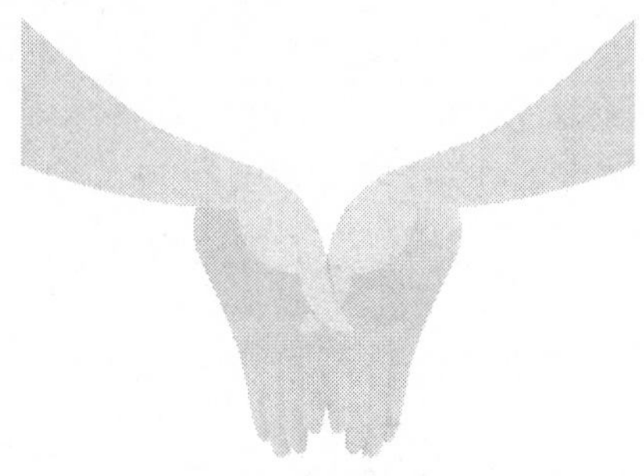

Lie flat on your back and gently massage the belly beginning on the right ovary area. Make gentle clockwise motions to warm the body. As you move toward the center of the body focus on lifting the uterus as you continue to make clockwise circles. Continue to the left ovary. As it feels comfortable you can increase the circle. You may also ask your partner to assist you and use a natural oil product like olive or avocado oil.

## Yoga Posture

Legs up on the wall diagram, (see Align the Spine.)

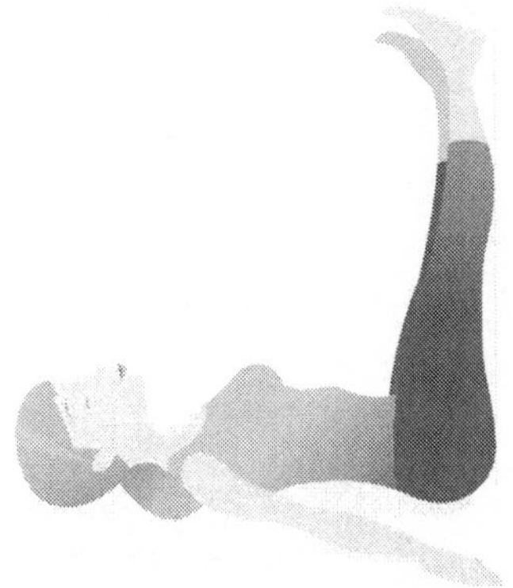

## A Mind-Body Perspective

"The average reproductive life span for a woman is about 30 years. Years ago, women didn't menstruate on the average until age 15 or 16. Today girls of 10 or 11 are already menstruating. Part of this is due to the overabundance of synthetic hormones in our diet. We are coming of age faster and going into menopause later. We should be able to prolong our reproductive health as well as longevity." [cxxiv]
— Randine Lewis

These days, many women are deciding to wait to have children, whether it is waiting for the "perfect" mate, a career choice or simply a change of heart later in life. In her best selling book,

*Women's Bodies, Women's Wisdom*, Dr. Christiane Northrup maintains, "Only 1/3 of women who defer childbearing into their mid- late thirties will have a problem with fertility. But fully two-thirds won't have any problem. And 50 percent of women in their early forties won't have a problem either." Dr. Northrup goes on to reveal that in different cultures, where age-related fertility is not recognized, women go on to conceive into their fifties and sixties.[cxxv] Even the National Center for Health Statistics is concurring, revealing that births over the age of 40 have doubled in the last decade.[cxxvi] The generalized distinction that women over the age of 35 will have trouble conceiving only contributes to a culture of fear. It then becomes worthy of consideration: just how are these labels impacting our fertility? Knowing that our thoughts impact our reality and physical form, it is essential to turn your attention to the miraculous ability of the body to recreate itself and return balance regardless of lab values and diagnostic terms.

**Dr. Kiltz Recommends**

With all the advances in assisted reproductive technologies, there are so many avenues that have opened up for women who want to have children later in life. Since there appears to be a decline in eggs over the years, I still like to encourage women to look at their options closely and move forward with the best course of action as soon as they are ready. Our culture tends to zone in on the problems associated with statistics, and it is worthy to note that our own perceptions have a lot to do with outcomes. As Dr. Northrup points out, there are women in many cultures who go on to have their babies well into their 40's and 50's. The concept of nurturing the fountain of youth by reducing stress and increasing blood flow to the ovaries can only support the egg quality. As we have discussed, lab values only depict part of the story. Miracles happen everyday, and we want to remain open to all possibilities.

## Endometriosis

### By definition…

Five million American women are currently living with endometriosis, though as many as 40% may experience no symptoms at all. Strangely, there are only 5 reported cases prior to 1921. Endometriosis occurs when tissue that normally grows within the uterus cavity begins to grow in other areas of the body, most commonly the pelvis and the bowel. In some cases, endometrial cysts implant in the fallopian tube obstructing the egg from implantation in the ovary, preventing ovulation. They can also act as a web of scar tissues, blocking the passage from the ovary to the fallopian tube and uterus. Though not overly common, endometriosis has been known to travel as far as the lungs, spine and the brain.

There seems to be a hereditary link with endometriosis, though not all women in the same family will manifest it, and the condition is likely depending on environmental factors. In fact, recent studies on monkeys have revealed a strong connection to dioxin exposure and the subsequent occurrences of Endometriosis and immune dysfunction. Further research is revealing an increased connection between endometriosis and a whole set of "atopic (allergic) diseases in these individuals and their families including allergies, food intolerances, asthma, eczema, and sometimes debilitating sensitivities to environmental chemicals such as perfumes, cigarette smoke, cleaning agents and others; a tendency to infections and mononucleosis; problems with Candida albicans; mitral valve prolapse; fibromyalgia and chronic fatigue immune dysfunction syndrome; and a greater risk for autoimmune disorders including lupus and Hashimoto's thyroiditis." [cxxvii]

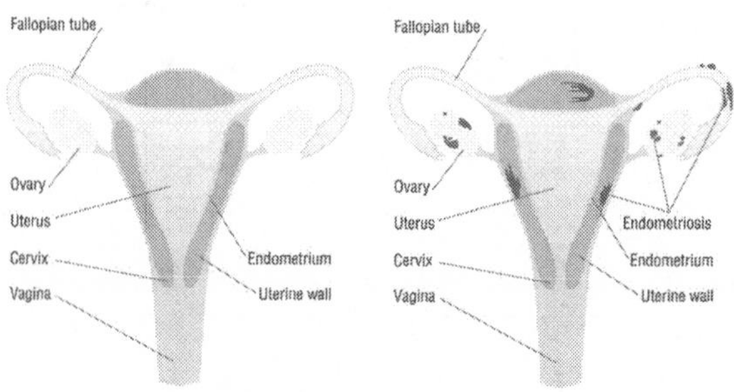

**Symptoms may include:**

- Painful period
- Pain at ovulation
- Cramps
- Pain during or after intercourse
- Pain during elimination
- Low back pain
- Spotting
- Bloating
- Diarrhea or constipation
- Fatigue
- Heavy bleeding
- Presence of auto-antibodies

**Western Medicine Testing and Treatments**

Endometriosis has four different levels of severity classified in The American Society for Reproductive Medicine's Revised Classification of Endometriosis: Stage I (Minimal) 1-5 points, Stage II (Mild) 6-15 points, Stage III (Moderate) 16-40 points, Stage IV (Severe) 40 points +. Diagnosis methodologies are the same in each case and are not based on level of pain, since many women have no symptoms whatsoever.

**Immune Response**

Blood tests - Elevated APA (antiphospholipid antibodies) indicate heightened autoimmune activity, which can both contribute to the original endometriosis and subsequent issues with fertility. High levels of these antibodies have also been linked to recurrent miscarriage, intrauterine growth, retardation and pre-enclampsia. The course of treatment for elevated APA is aspirin or low dose heparin.

Low levels of Beta-3, a substance required for healthy implantation, have also been linked to endometriosis, as have the presence of macrophages (natural killer cells) that may attack the sperm, egg or embryo.

**Physical**

Pelvic exam - an experienced physician may begin to suspect endometriosis after noticing endometrial nodules during the pelvic exam along with symptoms reported by the client. To verify the diagnosis, a laparoscopy is generally performed, where a sample of the tissue is removed to perform a biopsy of the tissue for confirmation.

**Surgeries**

A recent study of 172 women revealed that laparoscopic surgery performed on "infertile" women with even mild endometriosis did enhance fertility.[cxxviii]

Laparoscopy- the laparoscopy is the only way to

accurately diagnose endometriosis and gain a clear understanding of severity. During this procedure, a lighted scope is inserted through a tiny incision in the pelvis. Once the endometriosis is found, the surgeon may be able to remove most of the endometrial implants. If the endometriosis is more severe, a laparatomy may be performed, involving a larger incision and recovery time to fully remove the endometriosis. When the endometriosis is heavily lodged in the bowel cavity, part of the bowel may be removed and fused back together (a bowel resection).

**Medications and surgeries that impact fertility prospects:**

Some medications and surgeries used to treat endometriosis are not viable options for a woman looking to preserve her fertility and are primarily used by those whose chief intention is to reduce pain: Hysterectomy (removes reproductive organs), birth control (temporarily stops ovulation), progesterone-only shots (reduces estrogen to counteract development of endometrial tissue), GnRH agonists (causes menstruation to stop), and danazol (reduces estrogen by raising estrogens, can lead to menopause).

**A Chinese Medicine Perspective**

According to the Journal of Traditional Medicine, acupuncture has proven to have positive effects in treating pain in endometriosis, as well as improving blood circulation and regulating the endocrine system.[cxxix] This has been true in my practice where women most commonly report varying levels of pain combined with clotty, dark menses, low back pain and pre-menstrual cramping. When I look at their tongues I see a distinct purple or dark hue often alongside swelling. When I ask them to lift their tongue, the veins are commonly distended and purple. In Chinese medicine, endometriosis corresponds to the diagnosis of blood stasis with underlying spleen Qi deficiency, describing to coagulation and lack of free flow in the endometrial tissue and the autoimmune condition. My treatment strategy involves regulating the blood flow and calming inflammation to encourage healing, using acupuncture points Spleen 10, Spleen 8 and Spleen 6. Herbal medicine complements acupuncture by helping to restore balance in the hormone levels (reduce estrogen stores) and build up the immune system to eliminate endometrial tissue. The herbal formula Jia Wei Mo Jie Tang has shown promising impacts of reducing menstrual pain and decreasing levels of estradiol in women, and raising progesterone to support implantation. In a group of 125 women diagnosed with blood stasis (the Chinese definition of endometriosis) 80.4% experienced relief using Chinese herbal therapy over the Western medicine treatment, indomethacin, which showed no changes in estrogens or progesterone.[cxxx]

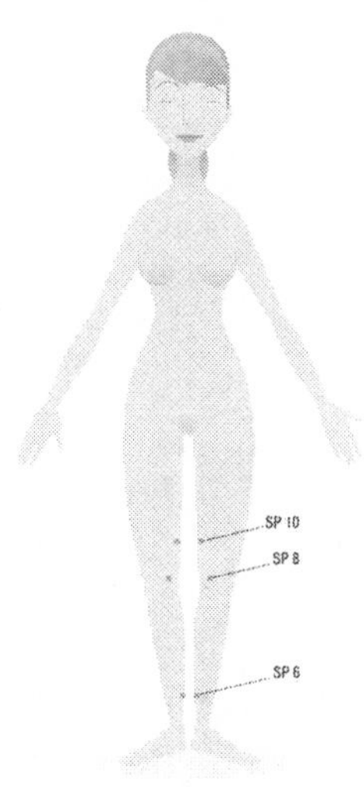


## Diet and Lifestyle Recommendations

Of primary importance for treating endometriosis is to reduce levels of inflammation and toxins that contribute to elevated estrogen levels. For this reason, endometriosis in particular warrants a vegetarian diet as most toxins in our 'standard American diet' are found in animal products (see chart). If you do eat animal products, be sure to choose organic. Follow the fertility diet guidelines (to support healthy immune function) along with these specific tips to help resolve endometriosis:

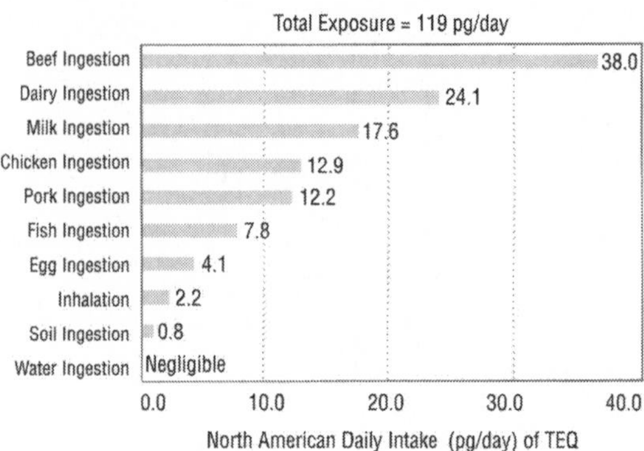


*The chart above depicts our daily exposure to environmental toxins.*[cxxxi]

- Avoid exposure to xeno-estrogens, environmental toxins that have been linked to estrogen dominance, include: insecticides parathion and DDT and its metabolites; herbicides; fungicides; plant and fungal estrogens; and industrial chemicals such as cadmium, lead, mercury, PCBs and dioxins[cxxxii]
- Avoid excess phytoestrogens; they have also been linked to conditions of estrogen dominance: Isoflavonoids - soybeans and soy products specifically the extracts: genistin, diadzein, and glycitin.
- Always choose organic forms of sustenance
- Eat an abundance of vegetables, whole grains and vegetable sources of protein

- Avoid foods with arachidonic acid: animal and dairy products, egg yolks and peanuts
- Include anti-inflammatory foods like dark leafy greens, omega-3 rich foods (salmon, mackeral, tuna)
- Eat cruciferous vegetables containing Diindolylmethane (DIM) (broccoli, brussels sprout, cabbage, collard greens, kale, horseradish, rutabaga, turnip, Chinese cabbage, cauliflower, broccoli rabe, daikon, bok choy, radish, spinach) which helps to reduce estradiol levels.
- Include sources of linoleic and alpha-linolenic fatty acids (evening primrose oil, pumpkin seed oil, black currant oil, linseed oil)
- Choose "blood stasis" reducing foods: abalone, beets, bilberry, brussels sprouts, chestnut, chili pepper, chive, crab, cucumbers, dark green vegetables, eggplant, evening primrose oil, fish and fish oil, hawthorn berry, kelp, lemon, lime, linseed oil, mustard leaf, nuts and seed oils, onion, peach, saffron, scallion, seaweed, spirulina, squid, sturgeon, turnips, vinegar.
- Use pads instead of tampons
- Partake in gentle movements including yoga, qi gong, walking and stretches that promote circulation and elicit the relaxation response

**Supplementation for Endometriosis**

-High quality prenatal vitamin/mineral that includes 1,000 mcg folic acid
-Fish oil (4,000 mg/day) - decreases inflammation, calms reactivity, increases uterine lining quality, overall support for hormonal balance, moderates NK cell activity
-OPC powder– decreases inflammation and increases circulation, helps to protect body's cells from free radicals damage
-Nattokanise – helps break up tissue and/or prevent clotting
-PABA (para-amino-benzoic acid) for immune related endometriosis

**Massage Recommendations**

ATMAM can be extremely soothing for the pain experienced from endometriosis, which is often caused by the body working too hard to shed the excess lining and adhesions attaching to the reproductive organs. It can also change the physiology of the body, help to heal endometriosis by realigning the uterus, aligning the spine to ensure no arterial blood flow is being cut off, and dealing with any retrograde blood flow issues cost by misalignment or structural issues. It is believed that the lack of circulation to the pelvis has a direct relationship to the autoimmune reaction, which, once regulated, will notice the endometrial tissue as foreign and dissolve it. Oftentimes, after extensive treatment, anywhere between 2-6 weeks, women notice endometrial tissue passing. Castor oil massages performed along with vaginal steam baths are helpful in treating endometriosis.

How to perform a **castor oil massage:**

What you'll need:

- ¼ cup cold pressed castor oil
- 1 cotton cloth
- 1 heating pad or hot water bottle
- Plastic wrap to cover heating pad
- 1 towel

Soak cotton cloth in castor oil and cover heating pad or hot water bottle with plastic wrap. Place castor oil-soaked cloth on the heating source and hold on lower belly, (you may want to use a large towel to hold the heating pad in place.) During months that you are attempting conception, use this technique only during your period. Otherwise, repeat this process daily for the first month and every second day the following month.

**Yoga Posture**

Detoxify excess estrogen from the liver with twists in the follicular phase.

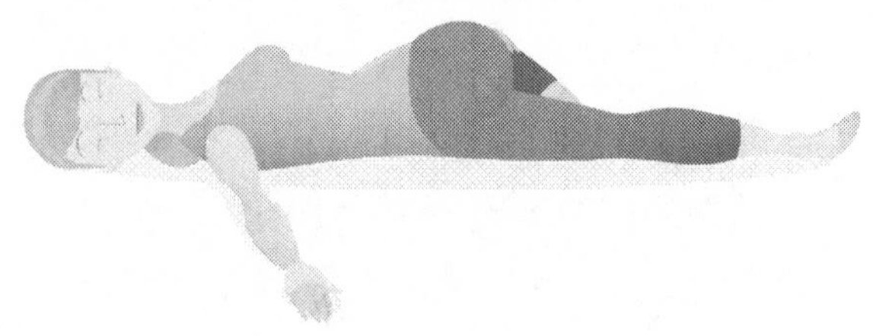

**A Mind-Body Perspective**

It is interesting to stop and realize that endometriosis barely existed prior to 1921, a time when we certainly had less information to process and less toxins in our natural environment. In *When the Body Says No*, Dr. Gabriel Mate delves into the field of psychoneuroimmunology in examining how our inability to speak up and say no to stress results in a variety of autoimmune conditions.[cxxxiii] Are we unable to say no to unreasonable expectations of what we can do in a day, in this lifetime? Dr. Northrup notes that endometriosis has also been referred to as the "career woman's disease," and "illness of competition," where "a woman's emotional needs are competing with her functioning in the outside world." She further concludes, "What would protect against the disease [endometriosis] would be business and personal environments that don't require a mental-emotional split." [cxxxiv]

**Self-Inquiry: Looking into our Environments**

Exercise: look at your calendar: are you doing at least one thing each day that brings you peace and calm and regenerates you? Begin to create balance in your everyday life.

Fung Shui: look at your work environment and find ways to bring peace and serenity into your environment: peaceful music, your favorite color? Favorite photos? Crystals?

**Dr. Kiltz Recommends**

It is wonderful to know that advances in laparoscopic surgery can restore fertility, especially immediately following treatment. Since endometriosis is shown to return after surgery, it is important to do the deeper work with the goal of permanently dissolving the endometrial tissue in your body. It's important that we each evaluate our life goals. Sometimes we get so carried away with the day to day, without even realizing that our internal and external commitments are imbalanced; we are grinding away each day and not refueling our deepest vitality. We can each do one thing each day to bring a sense of peace and calm into our lives. Consider the castor oil massage, acupuncture and yoga to illicit relaxation and calm our immune response. The more we can rid ourselves of environmental toxins in non-organic foods and xeno-estrogens (think plastics) the more we can reduce the prevalence of estrogen-dominant diseases like endometriosis. Load up on fresh antioxidant rich vegetables (especially broccoli and cauliflower) organic protein sources and whole grains topped with healthful evening primrose oil (rich in linoleic and alpha-linolenic fatty acids).

## Fibroids

### By definition…

Uterine fibroids are the most common growths of the female reproductive system. They are most often benign (non cancerous) tumors, composed of muscle tissue and develop within the uterus or attach to the uterine wall, varying in size (some up to 7 lbs). Fibroids appear in 1 out of 5 women of childbearing age and most often in women between the ages of 30 and 40 years old. The leading cause is excessive estrogen in the body that upsets the delicate balance of hormones and can lead to infertility.

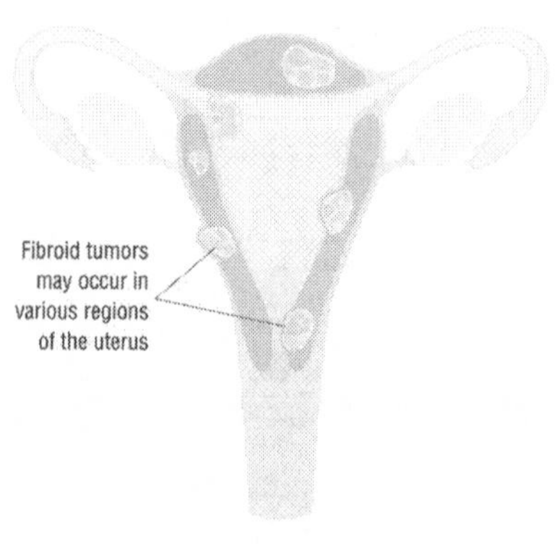

**Symptoms may include:**

- Bloating and gas
- Heavy bleeding during menstruation
- Long menstrual flow
- Bleeding between periods
- Frequent urination
- Cramping
- Severe abdominal/pelvic pain
- Pressure in lower abdomen
- Fullness
- Estrogen dominance
- Constipation
- Infertility

**Western Medicine Testing and Treatments**

When fertility is the goal, we want to use all of the treatments we can to avoid having a hysterectomy, of which 600,000 are performed each year.

Pelvic exams can sometimes reveal an irregularly shaped uterus or a mass in the pelvic region that warrant further investigation.

A pelvic ultrasound can give a more accurate picture of the size, number and shape of the fibroids.

An endometrial biopsy can take a piece of the tissue and confirm that the fibroid is benign.

Tissue can also be procured through a D&C.

A hysteroscopy uses a small camera inserted through the cervix to get a bird's eye view of fibroids and assess how their positioning may be impacting fertility. In the hysteroscopic resection, fibroids can be removed by use of a laser, wire or specialized electric knife without an incision. This can also be done through laparascopy, where an incision is made in the low abdomen. In the case that the fibroids are small, laparascopic surgery can remove fibroids through this incision. However, when fibroids are large, a laparoscopic myomectomy is often performed using an electric needle to destroy or shrink the masses through a small incision in the uterus.

A hysterosalpingography (hsg), where the dye is inserted into the uterus and fallopian tubes through the cervix to ensure there is a clear passage for reproductive function.

A myomectomy is performed to remove fibroids (non-cancerous growths in the uterus) from the uterus. It is done in conjunction with a laparoscopy and/or hysteroscopy. Fibroids may be detected during a hysterosalpingogram, causing your physician to recommend that they be removed. Fibroids can grow on the outside or inside of the uterus. A laparoscopy would be done to remove the fibroids on the outside of the uterus, as well as view and diagnose any additional issues with the ovaries, uterus or fallopian tubes. A hysteroscopy would be performed to remove the fibroids on the inside of the uterus and view the uterine lining or other issues that may be occurring in the uterus. A myomectomy is an out patient procedure that can last 1-3 hours, plus 1-2 hours of recovery time. Clients can return to work within a week.

Embolization is a procedure used under general or local anesthesia to shrink fibroids by cutting off their blood supply. Plastics inserts are inserted through a catheter in the groin into the blood vessels that supply flow to uterus, thereby reducing the size of the masses sometimes by half.

**Medications**

Gonadotropin releasing hormone (GnRH) (Depo Leuprolide or Lupron) works by reducing estrogen over a period of 3 months to shrink the fibroid. Complications include decreasing estrogen to the point of menopause, and also the possibility that the fibroid continues to grow once treatment stops.

RU-486 (mifepristone) has been shown to shrink fibroids in half and does not have the same side effects observed in the low estrogen consequences of GnRH.

Basic pain relievers (anti-inflammatories) like ibuprofen are often prescribed to counteract pelvic pain.

**A Chinese Medicine Perspective**

Sometimes women who have fibroids notice that they have an expanding waist and have to go up in clothing size before they realize a fibroid is the cause. From a Chinese medicine perspective, any accumulation in the pelvis will carry the similar diagnosis of blood stasis, usually with an underlying Spleen Qi deficiency. While cysts generally involve more pelvic pain, those experiencing fibroids usually report a heavier blood flow. The treatment strategy is to regulate the blood flow using the same acupuncture points as in endometriosis: acupuncture points Spleen 10, Spleen 8 and Spleen 6. Herbal formulas that help to dissolve cysts and fibroids generally include cinnamon and poria that help to move stagnant blood with Zi Gong Xue. A study recorded on The Fertile Soul website reveals a study where traditional Chinese herbs for blood stasis--along with any underlying pattern presented--were used to treat 223 cases of uterine fibroids. Of this group, fibroids shrunk or fully disappeared in 72% along with accompanying symptoms.[cxxxv]

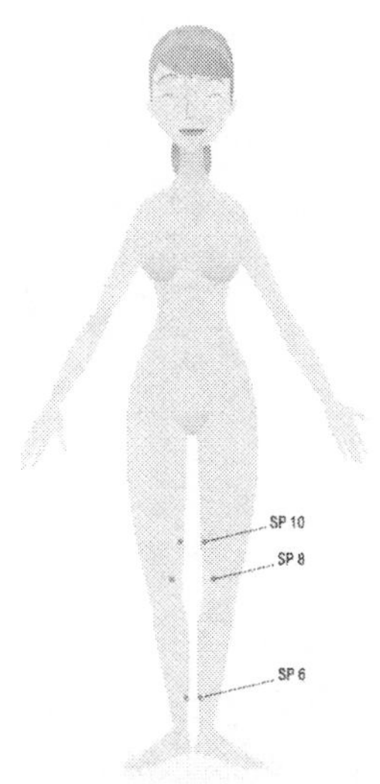


## Diet and Lifestyle Recommendations

Alongside the general guidelines for fertility, eating to reduce fibroids has some similar treatment goals to endometriosis. The goal is to lower estrogen dominance by adopting an all-organic, mostly vegetarian menu and reducing blood stagnation. It is also important to counteract heavy blood loss and potential anemia with iron supplements and/or foods. Since fibroids can also cause constipation, tips for improving digestion are included.

- If you are experiencing heavy bleeding, consume iron rich foods: dark leafy greens (spinach, kale, collard), dried fruit (prunes and raisins), mollusks (oysters, clams and scallops), bean lentils, chickpeas and artichokes

- Avoid xeno-estrogens in the environment like insecticides parathion and DDT and its metabolites; herbicides; fungicides; plant and fungal estrogens; and industrial chemicals such as cadmium, lead, mercury, PCBs and dioxins
- Avoid excess phytoestrogens. They have also been linked to conditions of estrogen dominance in isolated soy extracts
- Go organic
- Include anti-inflammatory foods like dark leafy greens, omega-3 rich foods (salmon, mackeral, tuna)
- Eat Diindolylmethane (DIM) containing cruciferous vegetables (broccoli, brussel sprouts, cabbage, collard greens, kale, horseradish, rutabaga, turnip, Chinese cabbage, cauliflower, broccoli rabe, daikon, bok choy, radish, spinach), which helps to reduce estradiol levels
- Include sources of linoleic and alpha-linolenic fatty acids (evening primrose oil, pumpkin seed oil, black currant oil, linseed oil)
- Drink milk thistle, chamomile and yogi detox tea
- Choose "blood stasis" reducing foods: abalone, beets, bilberry, brussel sprouts, chestnut, chili pepper, chive, crab, cucumbers, dark green vegetables, eggplant,

evening primrose oil, fish and fish oil, hawthorn berry, kelp, lemon, lime, linseed oil, mustard leaf, nuts and seed oils, onion, peach, saffron, scallion, seaweed, spirulina, squid, sturgeon, turnips, vinegar.

## Constipation relieving choices

- Eat lots of high fiber foods (leafy greens, whole fruits, brown rice, oats, legumes and beans)
- Start your day with a hot cup of water with lemon to cleanse your palette.
- Limit low fiber foods (meat, cheese, butter and sugar)
- Drink lots of room temperature water to help digest fiber
- Get some movement each day to keep your digestion flowing

## Supplementation for Fibroids and Cysts

- High quality prenatal vitamin/mineral that includes 1000 mcg folic acid
- Fish oil - decrease inflammation, calms reactivity, increase uterine lining quality, overall support for hormonal balance, moderates NK cell activity
- OPC powder– decreases inflammation and increases circulation, helps to protect body's cells from free radicals damage
- Nattokanise – helps break up and/or

prevent clotting
- Enzymes

**Massage Recommendations**

Massage can be used to detoxify the body of excess estrogen, as well as helping to shrink and reduce the presence of uterine fibroids. Along with restoring proper alignment and blood flow, the massage is energetically a form of clearing house both physically and emotionally. While fibroids, like endometriosis, benefit from castor oil massages and vaginal steambaths, the specific technique of ATMAM has been used since ancient times. ATMAM helps to resituate the uterus which may have become distorted from the fibroids, to restore circulation to the uterus, to improve lymphatic drainage, and to decrease the formation of scar tissue--all the while reducing pain. Maya Abdominal Massage trained therapists as well as some Chinese medicine practitioners perform uterine massage. Self-massage is recommended between sessions.[cxxxvi]

## Yoga Posture

Twists to detoxify the liver

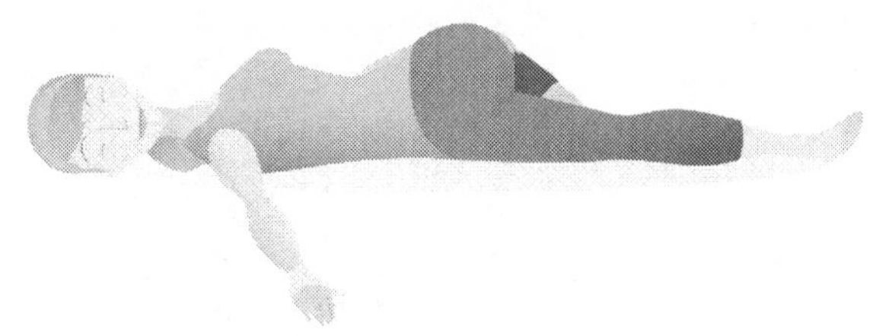

Note: Avoid practicing during your period. That might further dilate the blood vessels, causing heavier bleeding.

## A Mind-Body Perspective

The growth of a fibroid may be an indication of a creative block, according to medical intuitive Carolyn Myss. In her experience, she has noticed that fibroids are "often associated with conflicts about creativity, reproduction, and relationships" and may be indicating "creativity that has never been birthed in the world-dead-end life, jobs and relationships that are going nowhere."[cxxxvii] We all run into roadblocks from time to time, but most of us are conditioned to plough through without stopping to acknowledge what in our lives may not be contributing to our highest good.

Exercise from *Love and Infertility*: "The Dreams

List" [cxxxviii] with the intention of moving the feeling of constriction to revive creativity:

"If I had unlimited time, talent and money and support from my family, here is a list of all the things I would do with my life for the next twelve months."

Give yourself as much time as you need to brainstorm everything you would do. Once complete, choose your top three goals to complete in the coming year.

**Dr. Kiltz Recommends**

Fibroids are very common and believed to be responsible for fewer than 2% of infertility related cases. There are many options for removing fibroids, but alongside surgeries or medications, I recommend taking advantage of tried and true methods for shrinking and absolving fibroids on your own. Diet is a simple way to begin cutting out excess estrogens over time that will benefit you immensely, since estrogen dominance is not only linked to fertility issues, but also cancers. Massage is relaxing, and it helps detoxifies your body. If you can find a practitioner that is knowledgeable in the area of Uterine Fibroid massage, then by all means, set up an appointment and learn how to do it on your own time. If not, consider doing the castor oil massage that is helpful in restoring circulation and minimizing adhesions in the pelvis. As with every condition that involves stagnancy, the more you move your body and rid yourself of excess weight (that stores estrogen) the better off you will be. Find movement you love, and practice yoga twists to detoxify your body.

## Recurrent Miscarriage

### By definition…

Miscarriage is defined as the loss of a pregnancy prior to 20 weeks. An estimated 20% of all pregnancies end in miscarriages, and in many ways, it is nature's way of releasing a pregnancy that would not result in a healthy baby. Most women will go on to have a healthy pregnancy after the first loss, and the chances of conceiving begin to decline based subsequent miscarriages. Recurrent miscarriage is the spontaneous loss of three or more consecutive pregnancies experienced by 1 in 100 women.[cxxxix]

### Possible causes of recurrent miscarriage include:

- Chromosomal or genetic issues (up to 50%)
- Auto-immune disorder- antiphospholipid syndrome (APS)
- Hormonal causes: luteal phase defect (low progesterone during implantation), PCOS (high levels of androgens), diabetes (blood

sugar issues)
- Structural abnormalities in the uterus
- Incompetent cervix
- Age (after the age of 35 the chance of miscarriage increases)
- Infection
- Male factor
- Unexplained causes (50% of cases do not have a direct correlation of cause)

**Western Medicine Testing and Treatments**[cxl]

**Chromosomal genetic issues**

These affect 3-5 in 100 of those with recurring miscarriage.

When the DNA of two people comes together to create a third, an abnormality in the chromosomes of one or both of the parents may contribute to recurrent miscarriage. Genetic factors contribute to approximately 50% of all recurring miscarriages, with the most common abnormalities being: autosomal trisomies (22.3 percent), followed by monosomy X (8.6 percent), triploidy (7.7 percent) and tetraploidy (2.6 percent).[cxli]

**Inherited blood conditions** referred to as thrombophilia, including MTHFR and Factor V Leiden, can lend increased risk of blood clotting. Having this condition does not mean a blood clot will develop, and there are treatments (medications and vitamins) used prior to conception and during pregnancy to reduce coagulation: aspirin, 81 mg/d, folic acid, interferon, 4 mg/d, and heparin, 7,500 U SC twice daily.[cxlii]

An **embryo toxicity assay (ETA)** is sometimes performed to assess whether any circulating factors in the blood might be toxic to a growing fetus. This test is performed by using the woman's blood sample to create a culture for growing mouse embryos, and may reveal any toxicity to determine the cause of recurring miscarriage, though research is currently lacking.

A complete **karotyping profile** of both parents is helpful in diagnosing a genetic cause of recurring miscarriage. Fecal matter (from the embryo or fetus) may also be tested to determine what chromosomal abnormality may have caused the miscarriage. If abnormalities appear, a genetic counselor can guide you on your options.

**Pre-implantation genetic diagnosis and screening** prior to implantation via IVF will help to determine whether the fetus is viable according to chromosomal integrity.

**Autoimmune factor** - affects 15 in 100 of those with recurring miscarriage.

Our bodies utilize **antibodies** to fight off infection. When women have recurring miscarriages, it is prudent to test for lupus anticoagulant and anticardiolipin. Finding antiphospholid antibodies (aPL) indicates a correlation between the miscarriage and an autoimmune reaction, where the body views the developing fetus as an invader and attacks the tissue (also called an alloimmune reaction). Tests should be repeated twice in a period of six to eight weeks to ensure accuracy.

**Treatment for aPL antibodies** includes **low dose aspirin** and **heparin injections** in early pregnancy to prevent miscarriage and has been shown to help increase live births to seven in ten, compared with four in ten without treatment. Steroids have also been used, but carry more side effects and risks compared to aspirin and heparin.

**Immunotherapy** lacks research to show that there is a positive correlation with resolving recurrent miscarriage. One study showed that both IVIG and paternal leukocyte injections didn't show any benefits in preventing miscarriage.[cxliii] Treatments like third party donor cell immunization and trophoblast membrane infusion and intravenous immunoglobulins also appear to have no benefit in preventing miscarriage, according to the Royal College of Obstetricians and Gynecologists.

**Intralipids**

New research has suggested that women who have experienced recurrent miscarriages or multiple failed IUI or IVF cycles (as a result of natural killer cell activation) may benefit from the use of intralipids. Intralipids are synthetic and made from 1.2% egg yolk phospholipids, 10% soybean oil, 2.25% glycerin and water. It is administered through an IV 4-7 days before embryo transfer or insemination. Natural killer cells are regulated by the immune system. In women who have autoimmune issues, the natural killer cells can react abnormally to an implanting embryo, treating it as an invading cell and signaling for the body to attack it. Studies have found that intralipids can help to deactivate the natural killer cells, allowing the embryo to implant on the uterine wall and grow normally. Intralipids are re-administered 4-5 weeks following a positive pregnancy test, to keep the natural killer cells deactivated until the pregnancy can override the signals being sent by the immune system.

Intralipids (approximately $100 per administration) are far less expensive than Intravenous Immunoglobulin (IVIG) (approximately $2000 per administration), and initial studies show comparable efficacy for deactivation of natural killer cells and pregnancy rates. Intralipids are well tolerated by clients with few side effects and are created synthetically, unlike IVIG, which is a blood product. It takes about an hour and a half to two hours for the intralipids to be administered through the IVF.

For more information about intralipids call CNY Fertility Center or ask one of our nurses if you are a candidate, at your next appointment.

**Hormonal Imbalances**

Several hormonal conditions have been linked to recurrent miscarriage and treatment varies for each.

Note: Diabetes and thyroid issues can lead to miscarriage, though generally not recurrent miscarriage, since they can be treated and monitored.

**Polycystic Ovaries** affect just under 50% of women with recurrent miscarriage.

Women with PCOS have abnormally high levels of male hormones, androgens and high LH levels, which may disturb the perfect balance needed for healthy implantation. *(See PCOS section for treatment options).*

**Luteal Phase Defect** affects just under 25-60% of woman with recurrent miscarriage.

When there is insufficient progesterone in the luteal phase, it is more difficult to sustain pregnancy. Supplementation with progesterone creams or medications may help. *(See Luteal Phase Defect for treatment options)*

**Hyperprolactinarmia**- there is conflicting evidence that indicates an overproduction of prolactin may contribute to miscarriage.

**Structural abnormalities in the uterus** - affects just under 2-37 out of 100 women with recurrent miscarriage.

A **pelvic ultrasound** can visually access shape of the reproductive organs, while a hysterosalpingography (hsg) where the dye is inserted into the uterine cavity and fallopian tubes via the cervix can give a more specific view of any blockages or grades of severity in womb abnormalities. Small variations in structure are not believed to have an impact, where more serious abnormalities seem to contribute to miscarriage.

An **incompetent cervix** is more of a functional issue than a structural issue where the cervix opens too early on and stops the pregnancy. If your doctor deems it in the best interest of you and the baby, a procedure called a cerclage may be performed, where the cervix is stitched, in an attempt to prevent miscarriage.

**Infections** that enter the bloodstream may cause complications in pregnancy. The most common infection known to cause second trimester miscarriage and early delivery is bacterial vaginosis (BV). BV can be treated successfully with antibiotics.

Male factor- poor sperm health may contribute to recurrent miscarriage by impacting the health and viability of the embryo in the initial conception. A sperm analysis is important alongside any female fertility tests.

**Tests to Order: Recurrent Miscarriage**

- Full blood count
- Blood group
- Thyroid function tests
- Blood sugar
- Karyotyping
- Hormonal profile –LH,FSH,T1,PRL,DHEAS
- LA and ACA IgG and AgM
- Thrombophilia screen
- Transvaginal sonography
- Hysteroscopy
- Hsg
- Thyroid peroxidase antibody
- Autoantibody screen
- Total homocysteine
- Rubella status
- Free androgen index
- SHBG
- Male partner- Semen analysis-look for OAT and pyospermia

## A Chinese Medicine Perspective

Chinese medicine often looks at recurrent miscarriage through the lens of immune issues causing difficulty in implantation. The most common symptoms of an immune-related miscarriage are "feeling pregnant" and having the symptoms disappear, night sweats, a slight infection or flu-like symptoms in the luteal phase, anxiety, and BBT chart that shows a dip in the middle of the cycle without rise in temperature.

The most common Chinese medicine diagnosis is Spleen Deficiency with varying levels of Heat and Blood Stasis. The treatment strategy is to "lift the Spleen Qi" and calm the fetus, while lessening any reactivity in the immune response to ensure uterine lining is hospitable to implantation. The acupuncture points of choice include Stomach 25, Kidney 16, Liver 8, Du 20, Stomach 36 and Ren 12, adding Spleen 10 when blood stasis is present, and LI 11 when heat is present. Some of the most common formulas used for recurrent miscarriage are Dan gui and peony (Dan gui Shao Yao San). With blood stasis, cinnamon and Peoria are good choices.

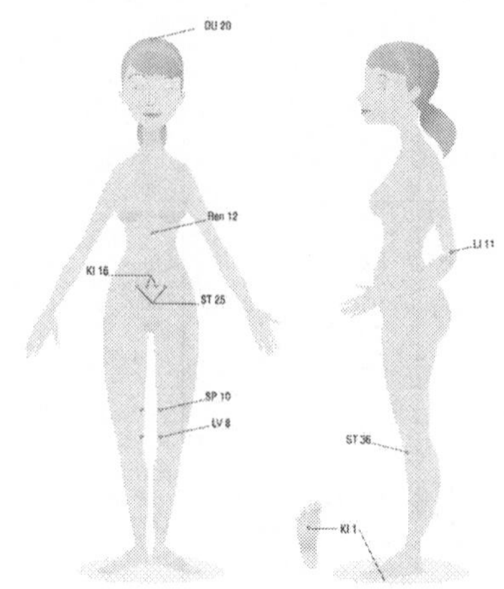


## Diet and Lifestyle Recommendations

In addition to the eating for fertility guidelines, supplement your diet with:

- Additional Folate: researchers have found higher homocysteine levels in women with a history of recurrent miscarriage.[cxliv] On top of folic acid supplements, eat plenty of legumes, lentils, chickpeas, collard greens, papaya, peas, asparagus, broccoli, strawberries and oranges.
- Nourishing simple meals like soup, grain, vegetables, and lean protein sources; add cut up dried kombu and wakame to dishes slowly simmered in water to soak up healthy minerals.
- Quit smoking, which has been correlated

with twice the incidence of miscarriage.

- Cut out caffeine: Kaiser Permanente Research shows the equivalent amount of caffeine in two cups of coffee increases your chance for miscarriage.[cxlv]
- Build up your deepest reserves with adequate rest, relaxation, meditation and breath work.
- Consume chlorophyll-rich foods to replenish your reproductive function: asparagus, bell peppers, broccoli, Brussels sprouts, green cabbage, celery, collard greens, green beans, green peas, kale, leeks, green olives, parsley, romaine lettuce, sea vegetables, spinach, Swiss chard, and turnip greens.
- Reduce heat with these foods: asparagus, bamboo shoot, banana, egg whites, clam, eggplant, elderflower, grapefruit, lemon, lettuce, melon, millet, mung beans, bean sprouts, peppermint, potato, salt, tofu, watermelon, wheat and by avoiding alcohol, red meat, chocolate, refined sugar, tobacco
- Gentle exercise: with recurrent miscarriage, it's important to choose activities that replenish the body like tai chi, walking and yoga.

**Supplementation for recurrent miscarriage and immune issues**

1. High quality prenatal vitamin/mineral that

includes 1000 mcg folic acid
2. Fish oil (4000 mg/day) – decrease inflammation, calms reactivity, increase uterine lining quality, overall support for hormonal balance, moderates NK cell activity
3. Baby Aspirin – increases blood flow and decreases inflammation
4. OPC powder– decreases inflammation and increases circulation, helps to protect body's cells from free radicals damage
5. Wobenzym - enzymes to help decrease autoimmune reactivity
6. PABA – indicated for MTHFR - stimulates production of folic acid
7. Blue Green Algae – neutralizes immune reactivity in body
8. Vitamin C – boosts immune system and helps to correct luteal phase defect
   Nattokanise - helps break up adhesions and works to prevent clotting
9. Additional Folic Acid in the form of 5-Methyltetrahydrofolate

**Massage Recommendations**

There are a couple theories regarding the causes of recurrent miscarriage in Arvigo Maya Massage theory.[cxlvi] The first belief is that the hormonal feedback loop is not functioning optimally, and therefore not preparing the body for pregnancy. The second thought is that if the blood supply to the uterus is inadequate, the growing fetus will not receive adequate nutrition. Light reflexology and gentle relaxation massages are the best forms of bodywork for recurrent miscarriage. Avoid overly detoxifying massages that can drain the system and release too many toxins into the system.

**Yoga Posture**

Deep belly breathing to connect the heart and uterus/ open the conception vessel.

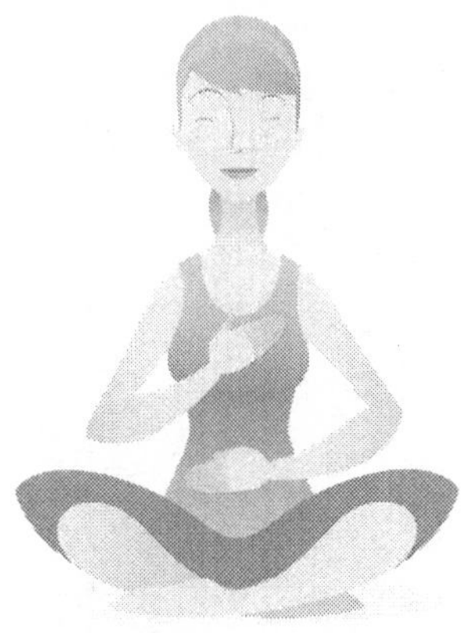

**A Mind-Body Perspective**

Oftentimes, our society does not acknowledge the tremendous grief that accompanies the loss of a baby, not to mention recurring losses of babies in utero. The emotion of grief is strong, and when repressed, can lead to numbness and emotional distress. It is commonly known that there are 5 stages of grief: denial, anger, bargaining, depression and acceptance. Each stage must be fully embraced before we reach the final stage of acceptance, and pretending will not help in this scenario *(See Lisa Stack's article in Shift from Mind to Heart)*. It may also feel helpful to perform your own grief ceremony, either on your own or with a group of friends. A suggested format would be to do a brief meditation and connect with the unborn baby, then light a candle of remembrance, and allow yourself to feel whatever comes up. Dr. Christiane Northrup believes miscarriage is a sign that your body may be fighting against itself and indicates an importance to nurture yourself above all else.[cxlvii] Clairvoyant, Walter Makichen cautions his clients to realize that a miscarriage rarely indicates that a conception contract has been broken, and more often means that the spirit baby is still overwhelmed by the challenges that our world has, and is not ready to enter the body.[cxlviii]

## Dr. Kiltz Recommends

Having a miscarriage is physically and emotionally devastating. The most common question I hear is "What could I have done differently?" There is so much unknown about the cause of miscarriage and why certain pregnancies take and others do not. Through testing we can learn what can be done differently the next time. The most important thing you can do is to nurture yourself. Allow yourself to experience the grief that is real, and don't be surprised if you experience emotional swings while your hormones are rebalancing. Be gentle with yourself. Begin to replenish your deepest reserves with acupuncture and massage. Maya Abdominal Massage is an extremely healing practice in the instance of miscarriage, as it can help to release patterns of grief that are stored in the belly.

## Luteal Phase Defect

### By definition…

The luteal phase is the time between ovulation and the first day of your period. When impregnation occurs, it is during this time that the fertilized egg will travel to the uterus via the fallopian tube for implantation. The luteal phase generally lasts 14 days, but can range anywhere between 10 to 17 days. A luteal phase less than 12 days indicates low progesterone levels, leading the uterine lining to break down, causing menstrual bleeding, inability to implant and the potential for recurrent miscarriage.

### Symptoms may include:

- Low progesterone levels (less than 14 ng/ml after ovulation)
- Thin endometrial lining

- Pre-menstrual spotting
- Short luteal phase
- Fatigue
- Cold (as seen by the lack of rise in temperature on the BBT chart after ovulation)
- Vaginal discharge
- Thyroid imbalance
- Hyperlactomenia (abnormally high levels of prolactin)

**Western Medicine Testing and Treatments**

There are several causes of luteal phase defect, each with its own treatment strategy:

1. **Poor follicular development-** in the case where FSH is low or there may be a lack of response in the ovaries, the follicle development will be inadequate, impacting the quality of the corpus luteum and subsequently the release of progesterone necessary to allow a fertilized egg to implant.
2. **Inadequate corpus luteum-** other than beginning with poor follicular development, the corpus luteum sometimes ceases to create the necessary levels of progesterone to sustain an adequate lining.
3. **Thin uterine lining-** can persist even with adequate follicular and corpus luteum development. Implantation may fail in this

case.

**Endometrial Biopsy** is one of the best ways to accurately diagnose LPD. In this procedure, an endometrial sample is gathered two days before the beginning of a woman's cycle. The lab technician assigns a date to the sample and if it is consistent with the actual date, then a woman is "in phase." However, when the dates do not match, indicating the woman is "out of phase" consistently in two separate samples, the diagnosis of LPD is given.

### Medications

Progesterone therapy is the general course of treatment to treat inadequate production of progesterone from the corpus luteum. In the case of low follicular stimulation Clomid, or a similar ovulatory drug, is used to stimulate ovulation to encourage follicles to mature properly.

### A Chinese Medicine Perspective

When a women walks into our office with luteal phase defect, she typically reports some of the most common signs associated with luteal phase defect including spotting, a short cycle, and an inability to get pregnant or recurrent miscarriage. When we begin to examine the client, we almost always notice one of two patterns. In the first case, we see a weak kidney and spleen pulse and a pale, slippery and puffy tongue with a slowly declining BBT after ovulation. For these clients, the treatment strategy is to "warm" the yang and boost spleen Qi to help calm the fetus, thereby preventing miscarriage. Key acupressure points are St 36, Du 20 and Ki 7 alongside herbal formulas with ginseng and astragalus. In the second case, luteal phase defect may be resulting from too much heat in the blood, resulting in a red tongue (or dots) with a high temperature that plummets with onset of spotting or menses. In this case, the goal is to clear excess heat and nourish yin to support healthy implantation. The acupuncture points used are Li 11, K3, Li 2, along with free and easy wanderer plus or in the case of "deficient heat," rheumania and scofleuria. To confirm the diagnosis, we ask the client to chart their BBT over a period of 3 months to see how the treatments impact their temperatures after ovulation. Ideally, we want to see the temperature building after ovulation for at least 12 days or more, indicating adequate progesterone and uterine lining. Generally treating luteal phase can take anywhere from 3-6 months. Sometimes women opt to supplement with progesterone cream during the second half of their cycle.

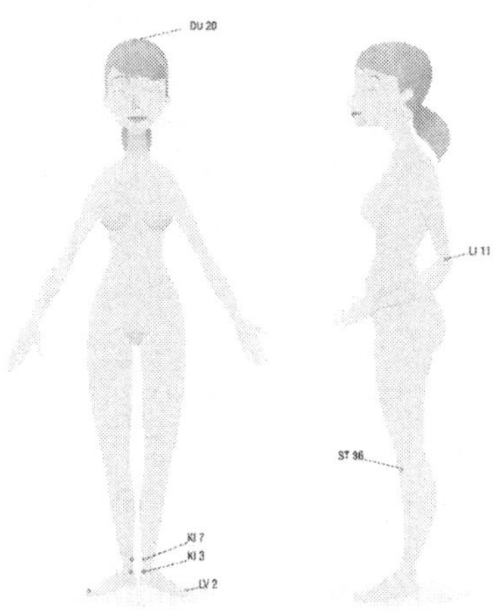


## Diet and Lifestyle Recommendations

Follow the fertility diet guidelines, paying special attention to:

1. Eat a colorful array of fruits, vegetables, grains, proteins and fats to ensure you are getting all of your nutrients
2. B vitamins, especially B6, and magnesium support optimal progesterone production. You can get optimal amounts by taking a quality supplement and enjoying B6 rich foods[cxlix]

- **B6 sources**: avocado, bananas, yeast extract, dried brewer's yeast, wheat bran, wheat germ, oat flakes, sardines, mackerel, beef, poultry, brown rice, cabbage, molasses, free range eggs

- **Magnesium sources**: pumpkin seeds, spinach, Swiss chard, soybeans, salmon, sunflower seeds, sesame seeds, halibut, black beans.

**Supplementation for Luteal Phase Defect**

- High quality prenatal vitamin/mineral that includes 1000 mcg folic acid
- Fish oil – decrease inflammation, calms reactivity, increase uterine lining quality, overall support for hormonal balance, moderates NK cell activity
- Vitamin C - boosts immune system and corrects luteal phase defect

**Yoga Posture for hormonal balance**

Alternate Nostril Breathing to Balance yin (estrogen) and yang (progesterone) and calm the nervous system.

Sitting cross-legged, allow the left hand to rest on the left knee. Lift the right hand and place the thumb on the right nostril. Inhale through the left nostril and close with the ring finger, hold for a moment and then release the thumb, exhaling. Inhale through the right nostril close with the thumb, hold and release the ring finger exhaling through the left nostril. Repeat, slowly allowing the body to relax.

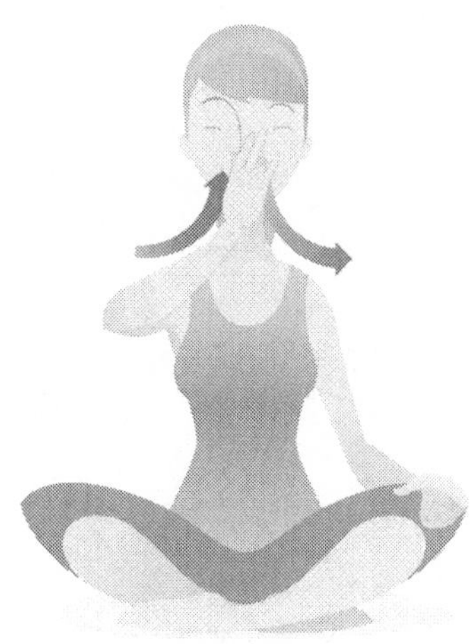

## Massage Recommendations

ATMAM is a wonderful way to increase the quality of the follicles in the first half of the cycle, leading to healthy corpus luteum and progesterone production. The Femoral massage is another technique that partners can do together, where the husband presses down on the woman's femoral artery for 30 seconds, stopping the blood from flowing. When the pressure is released, a surge of fresh blood rushes to the ovaries, nourishing the developing follicle. Massage done in partnership can also help to increase the bond between partners and stimulate the libido.

*Femoral Massage* by Randine Lewis, Ph.D., L.Ac., used with permission from The Fertile Soul

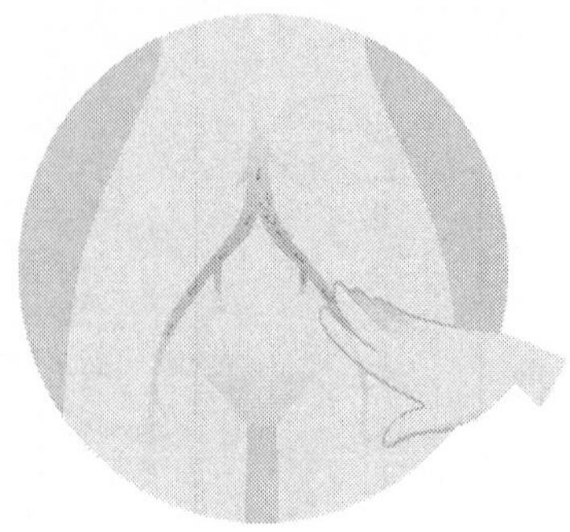

This exercise can be performed alone or with a partner, two times a day before ovulation. Repeat the exercise up to three times. The intention is to increase blood supply to ovaries and uterus.

1. Find the crease between your upper thigh and the trunk of your body.
2. Using your fingertips, locate the femoral artery (as in picture).
3. Find the pulsation and press down deeply into the artery until you feel the pulse stop.
4. Hold for 30-45 seconds and allow the blood flow to gather in the uterus and ovaries.
5. Release the pressure and resume natural flow. You will feel a warm rush as the blood returns down your leg.
6. Repeat on the opposite side.
7. Gently massage the belly in clockwise rotations lifting the uterus and ovaries.

## A Mind-Body Perspective

The sheer name of this diagnosis is something that needs to be reframed. The word "defect" implies a problem, when perhaps our body is simply flowing to a different rhythm and needs to be nurtured back to balance. Self-nurturing is first and foremost with any hormonal imbalance. What does your body need to feel most vital and alive? Are you feeding your cells with nourishing foods, replenishing exercise and positive vibrations? Simply becoming aware of the way our cycles flow with the energies of the moon can make us cognizant of our different needs at various times of the month. Please note that menstrual cycles vary among women and we are using the example of 28 days as a generalization below.

1. Follicular Phase (Day 1-14)- a time to be outgoing, social while deeply nourishing our baseline energies with equal rest and equal play
2. Ovulation (Day 11-21)- the sexiest time of the month, communication, connection and union are paramount
3. Luteal Phase (Day 14-28)- a time to retreat, relax and regenerate. Allow the activities from the beginning of the month to unfold and manifest without force.
4. Menstrual Phase (Day 21-7)- both before and during menses, we transform by shedding the old and making room for what

is new. A time of transformation and allowing ourselves to enter the cocoon and emerge as butterfly.

### Dr. Kiltz Recommends

Luteal phase defect usually responds well to treatment and can really benefit from a holistic approach that includes acupuncture, diet, massage and a high level of self-nurturance. The initial diagnosis, using the endometrial biopsy, is the best way to get an accurate picture of how far out of phase a woman is in her cycle. With that knowledge, we can assess what treatment strategy will work best and move forward. While progesterone cream offers an immediate solution, it is also possible to use herbs that encourage your body to create additional progesterone and supplement with magnesium and B6 vitamins and foods.

## Male Factor Infertility

### By definition…

Though infertility is often looked upon as a "female issue," nearly half of fertility problems can be attributed to the male. In order for conception to occur, sperm must be abundant in count, maintain a "normal shape" (morphology) and have the ability to move forward with speed to fertilize a women's egg (motility). About 40-50 percent of men who experience fertility issues have a varicocele- a varicose vein in the scrotum- that can cause swelling and interferes with the sperm production and testosterone levels, obstructing the vas deferens, causing blood to flow backwards to the scrotum, (retrograde ejaculation), which overheats affecting sperm quality. In some cases, CBAVD (congenital bilateral absence of the vas deferens) the tube that connects the sperm with the testes, is not properly developed, and though the condition has been present since birth, it goes undiagnosed until a man has issues with fertility. Other factors that can contribute to male factor fertility issues include environmental toxins, impotence, chemotherapy, duct obstructions, scarring from STD's, smoking nicotine or marijuana, alcohol consumption, and certain prescription drugs along with medical conditions like mumps or autoimmune disorders (anti-sperm antibodies).

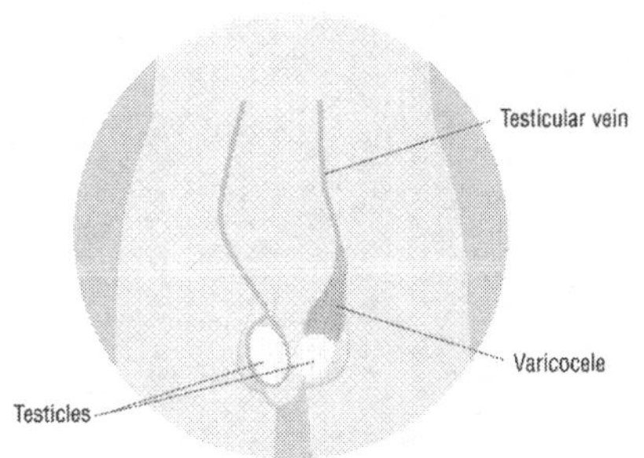

**Symptoms may include:**

- Swelling in scrotum
- High temperature
- Estrogen dominance
- Inability to conceive without known female factors

**Western Medical Testing and Treatments**

**Physical examination**. A visit to a urologist is most helpful for identifying the presence of a varicocele, a reversible condition that, once corrected, can re-establish fertility.

**The hormone panel** will show any discrepancy in levels that may be interfering with sperm production. Certain hormones may be replaced with medications, though hormone replacement is not used as often or as effectively with men.

**Antibody test** the presence of ANA antibodies may indicate that a man's body is hostile to his own sperm. In this case, sperm are seen as invaders and are attacked and destroyed. This can also happen when sperms enter a woman's vagina if the pH levels are not alkaline enough.

**Semen analysis** is one of the most important determinants to access the quality of a man's sperm. In this test, the man is directed to abstain from ejaculation for at least 72 hours, after which time he can provide a sample by masturbating into a sterile container. The sample must be evaluated within 2 hours to accurately gage count, morphology and motility.

- Deficient sperm count less than 20 million per milliliter.
- Motility: at least 50% with forward movement
- Less than 30 percent normal forms

**Testicular Biopsy** is a procedure used when a man is found to have very little or no sperm. The biopsy is a quick and relatively painless process when a small incision is made into each testicle to remove a piece of testicular tissue. The procedure is usually done with a local anesthesia. The biopsy is examined to ascertain the presence of sperm and any abnormalities in production or maturation. If sperm appears normal in the testicular biopsy, and yet did not appear in the semen sample, it is assumed that there is a blockage in the vas deferens and surgery is recommended.

**Genetic testing and karotyping** are used to rule out any pre-existing conditions that might impact the health of the sperm. Relevant conditions include: Klinefelter Syndrome, Cystic Fibrosis or Y Deletion. To support the diagnosis of CBAVD, men should be screened for the presence of a combination of a mutation known as R117H, and a specific variation in the CF gene known as the 5T allele.

**Medical treatments** have continued to evolve and can greatly increase a couple's chance of conceiving, despite limited sperm health. Some of the most common procedures include:

**IUI (Intrauterine insemination)** helps to increase the number of sperm that reach the fallopian tube and increase the chances of conception. In this procedure, a sperm sample is collected and injected into a woman's uterus. The procedure must be coordinated with the female's natural cycle, clomiphene citrate induced cycle, or gonatropin stimulated cycle. In the case of a natural cycle, ovulation predictor kits can be used to detect the LH surge; in gonatropin-induced cycles, HCG is injected when follicles are adequately developed to incite ovulation within 36 hours; clomiphene citrate is used to increase the number of mature follicles.

**IVF** in combination with **ICSI** has considerably higher rates for pregnancy with male factor (66% vs. 6-9% with IUI's). In the case of ICSI a single sperm is injected to fertilize the egg. This surpasses issues with sperm count and motility, allowing doctors to choose the healthiest of sperm even when sperm levels are undetectable (azoospermia). **TESE** is used in azoospermic men to retrieve testicular tissue and collect live sperm from the sample. Since very few can be collected in this way, ICSI is the only way for fertilization to occur.

These revolutionary techniques are so advanced that the success of the procedure becomes wholly dependent on the woman, since the male's issues are bypassed.

**Varicocele surgery** is usually performed under general anesthesia and involves a small incision in the scrotum to access the veins and redirect the blood flow by ligating the affected veins. These days, **varicocele embolization** has become more popular, because it avoids the use of anesthesia, incisions and sutures, so recovery time is significantly reduced. In this procedure, a catheter is inserted through the tiniest nick in the leg and guided up through the abdomen into the variococele. Using an x-ray to view the procedure, dye is inserted into the vein and embolizing substances like metal coils are used to block the flow of the vein.

**A Chinese Medicine Perspective**

When a man has a variocole or poor morphology, we will most often see signs of blood stasis demonstrated by a dark purple tongue. In supporting the resolution of a variocole and improving sperm's shape, our intention is to reduce inflammation and heat so sperm can generate properly. The best herbs to use are cinnamon and poria, along with the acupuncture points: Sp 10, 6 and Liver 3. To support healthy sperm count, motility and morphology, the overall treatment strategy is to increase blood flow to the reproductive organs through a combination of acupuncture and herbs. Motility issues indicate a lack of spleen Qi and or Kidney Yang, and low sperm count is also a deficiency in Spleen Qi and blood, both evidenced by a pale tongue. To improve motility and count, the herb Six Gentlemen is used in combination with the acupuncture points: St 36, Ki 7, Ren 3 and 4, which can support fluid movement and abundance.

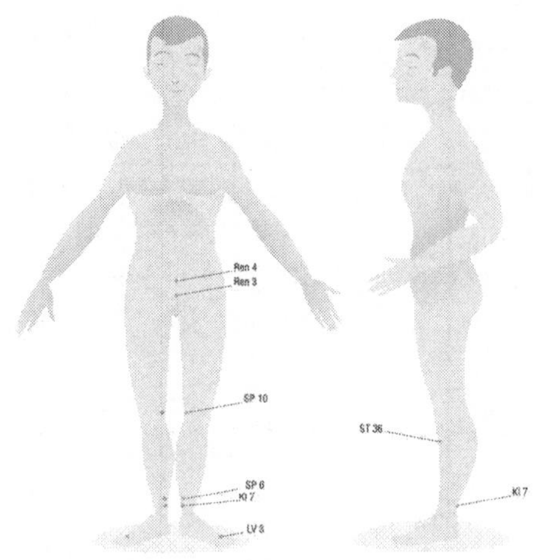


**Study: How Acupuncture Improves Sperm Production[cl]**

"In conjunction with ART or even for reaching natural fertility potential, acupuncture treatment is a simple, noninvasive method that can improve sperm quality. Further research is needed to demonstrate what stages and times in spermatogenesis are affected by acupuncture, and how acupuncture causes the physiologic changes in spermatogenesis. Our future aim is to strengthen our findings by enlarging the study group for more investigations." –Randine Lewis

## Diet and Lifestyle Recommendations

1. Get daily exercise, but avoid excessive biking- biking can cause impotence and lower sperm count due to pressure from the bike seat on nerves and blood vessels surrounding the scrotum.
2. Take time to relax each day- mental stress has been linked to lower sperm count. Meditating, reading or taking some time off work can regenerate your system and your sperm reserves.
3. Avoid excessive heat- avoiding saunas and hot tubs may be a good idea while trying to conceive. Exposure to excessive heat may reduce sperm count.
4. Boxers over briefs- briefs hold the testicles closer to the body causing the sperm to heat up and lower in count. Choosing boxer shorts keeps sperm at a more moderate temperature, which is preferable.
5. Avoid intoxicants including alcohol, marijuana and cigarettes- all intoxicants

affect the quality and quantity of the sperm. What you do today impacts your sperm in the next 10 weeks, so creating some healthy habits can reverse the impact of past habits.

6. In addition to the lifestyle habits listed above, eat a fresh, organic diet that includes the following nutrients: vitamin C, beta-carotene, vitamin E, selenium, vitamin B12, zinc, co-enzyme Q10, ginseng, flaxseed oil, omega 3, and wheat grass.
7. Follow a mostly alkaline diet: 70% alkaline, 30% acidic.

**High Alkaline Forming Foods:** string beans, banana, dandelion greens, dates, figs, prunes, raisins and swiss chard, almonds, asparagus, avocado, fresh beans, beets, black-berries, carrot, cranberries, chives, endive, sour grapes, kale, dried peach, persimmon, plum, pomegranate, raspberries, rooibos tea and spinach, agar, alfalfa, apple, fresh apricot, globe artichokes, bamboo shoots, snap beans, sprouted beans, most berries, broccoli, brussel sprouts, cabbage, cantaloupe, cauliflower, celery, cherries, chestnuts, chicory, coconut milk, collards, corn (when fresh), cucumbers, daikon, eggplant, escarole, garlic, ginger root, gooseberry, grapefruit, guava, horseradish (fresh and raw), kelp, kohlrabi, leek, lemon, lettuce, line, loganberry, mango, melons, raw, milk, millet, acidophilus yogurt and whey.

**High Acid Forming Foods:** alcohol, artichoke

root, barley, bread, buckwheat, caffeine, coffee, corn (when processed and not fresh), custards, drugs, most flours, ginger preserves, honey, lentils, pate, oatmeal, peanuts rice, rye grain, soy bred, soy noodles, sorghum, spaghetti, and other pastas, sugar cane, raw beets tobacco, walnut, wheat, dried beans, cashews, coconut, cranberry juice and concentrate, egg yolk, filberts, fruit jellies (canned jams, sulfured, sugared, dried), grapes, pasteurized milk products, dry peas, pecans, Damson plums, tofu, fries and water chestnuts.

## Supplementation for Male Factor Infertility

| | |
|---|---|
| Low Sperm Count | 1.High quality prenatal /mineral<br>2. OPC powder- decreases inflammation and increases circulation, helps to protect body's cells from free radicals damage<br>3. Vitamin C- improves sperm quality<br>4. Fish oil - decrease inflammation, overall support for hormonal balance |
| Poor morphology (varicocele) | 1. High quality vitamin/mineral<br>2. OPC powder- decreases inflammation and increases circulation, helps to protect body's cells from free radicals damage<br>3. Fish oil - decrease |

| | |
|---|---|
| | inflammation, overall support for hormonal balance<br>4. Milk thistle - cleanses liver, improves blood circulation and morphology |
| Poor motility | 1. High quality vitamin/mineral<br>2. OPC- decreases inflammation and increases circulation, helps to protect body's cells from free radicals damage<br>3. Fish oil - decrease inflammation, overall support for hormonal balance<br>4. CoQuinone- supports cellular energy production to improve motility |
| Prostate inflammation /pain | 1. High quality vitamin/mineral<br>2. Fish oil - decrease inflammation, overall support for hormonal balance<br>3. Saw Palmetto - decreases inflammation, pain or erectile dysfunction |

## Yoga for Male Factor Infertility

Sitting in butterfly posture with the soles of your feet touching, feeling the stretch through the groin as your inner thighs drop towards the earth. This posture helps with blood circulation.

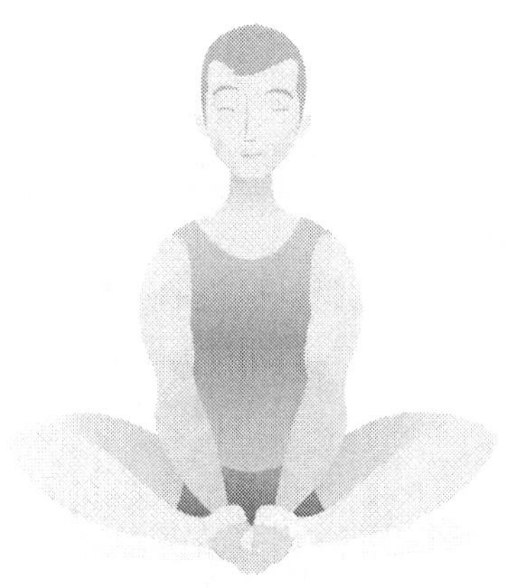

**Massage Recommendations**

According to Rosita Arvigo, creator of the Arvigo techniques of Maya Abdominal Massage, this type of massage helps the "drainage of the tubules from the testicles to prostate. This will eliminate the tendency of accumulation, concentration and hardening of the milky fluid exudates and thus prevent further pathology. The lymphatic drainage techniques will also be important. The lymphatic system needs to be cleared in preparation to receive the flow of stagnant fluids from the prostate. This will often result in milky urine for a few days which is a good sign of internal cleansing having taken place".[cli] Ice packs or placing the penis in cold water, alongside consistent massage of the scrotum are also recommended to help lower temperature, reduce inflammation and prevent swelling in the case of a varicocele.

## A Mind-Body Perspective

Male factor infertility can wreak havoc on a man's self esteem. The communication between the couple is paramount in preserving the relationship while enduring the stress of infertility. In *Love and Infertility: Survival Strategies for Balancing Infertility Marriage and Life*, by Kristen Magnacca, she offers strategies to help support each other without losing the love in your relationship. In this case, co-creating a fertility game plan with reflective listening to ensure you are both on the same page is so important. Issues of inferiority may present as grief, anger and confusion, and practicing reflective listening using the following strategies from *Love and Infertility: Survival Strategies for Balancing Infertility Marriage and Life* can help you from reacting prematurely and with an attacking nature.[clii]

**Recognize** the emotion boiling up beneath the words being spoken.

**Remind** yourself to listen with single focus and make eye contact to be fully present.

**Reflect** back the underlying feeling with an empathetic voice: "I hear you saying you feel…"

**Retreat** so they can acknowledge what you have said and feel their feelings or respond.

**Request** by inquiring whether or not your help is needed without assuming you need to find a solution. Sometimes people just need to feel and be heard.

### Dr. Kiltz Recommends

I always insist on seeing the couple in the first session because it is important to breakthrough the myth that infertility is a woman's issue. The journey to conception is a couple's affair and preliminary testing should be completed on both parties before a course of action is determined. Western medicine is so advanced in its technologies to reverse the common varicocele and ICSI rates of success are considerably higher than IUI. Consistent massage and acupuncture to reduce inflammation, heat and improve blood flow will support count, motility and morphology. Of course, where sperm is an issue, always boxers over briefs, avoid excessive heat and load up on antioxidant support.

## PCOS (Polycystic Ovarian Syndrome)

### By definition…

PCOS, also called Stein Leventhal Syndrome, is one of the leading causes of infertility. In PCOS, high levels of androgens lead to increased LH levels and low FSH levels that prevent follicles from developing, disrupting ovulation. Without ovulation, progesterone stops being produced and estrogen levels remain consistent. In "normal" ovulation, follicles develop in the ovaries, maturing over the course of the month until one mature egg is released. In the case of PCOS, eggs are trapped within follicles that become fluid-filled cysts. Each month, the hormonal imbalance prevents ovulation, resulting in swollen, cyst-filled ovaries, sometimes measuring the size of a grapefruit.

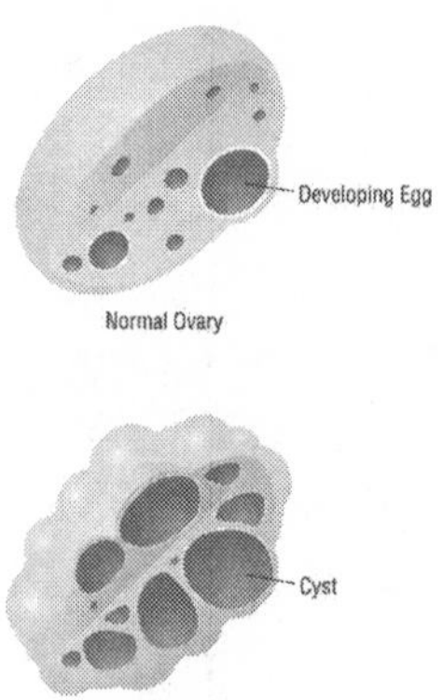


**Symptoms may include:**

- Amenorrhea (the absence of menstruation)
- Long menstrual cycles (more than 35 days between menses)
- Heavy bleeding
- Anovulation

- Weight gain and obesity
- Depression
- Insulin resistance and hyperinsulinemia (too much insulin)
- Diabetes
- Acne
- Hair loss
- Recurrent miscarriages
- Chronic pelvic pain
- Male sex characteristics: hirsutism (excessive facial hair, body hair), deepening voice, clitoral enlargement
- High lipid levels in bloodstream (cardiovascular risk)

**Western Medicine Testing and Treatments**

**Pelvic ultrasound** gives an image of the ovaries where a doctor can look for cysts, lesions and abnormalities that may lend to the diagnosis of PCOS.

**Fasting Biochemical Screen** will provide useful information about the client's insulin resistance scores, which is a determinant in the PCOS diagnosis.

**The Hormone Panel** for PCOS generally includes an SHBG test to determine levels of androgens, testosterone, LH and FSH. In PCOS testing, the LH:FSH ratio is used in the diagnosis. The ratio is usually close to 1:1, but if the LH is higher, it is one possible indication of PCOS.

**Additional blood tests:** Other disorders that produce hormone imbalances must be ruled out before PCOS can be diagnosed: hypothyroidism (an underactive thyroid that can't sort hormone concentrations), congenital adrenal hyperplasia (an excess or deficiency is sex hormones), hyperprolactinaemia (elevated prolactin).

**Medications**

**FSH** is injected in a procedure called ovarian hyper-stimulation to promote follicular growth and ovulation during an IVF cycle.

**Dexanethasone** is sometimes used to shrink cysts.

**Insulin regulators**, including metformin hydrochloride, pioglitazone hydrochloride and rosiglitazone maleate, are used to lower insulin levels that can help to restore ovulation.

**Surgeries:**

**Laparoscopy electrocauterization**: in this process a long thin tube with a camera is inserted into the pelvic cavity to look for any abnormalities and remove cysts and lesions by electric pulse.

**Ovarian drilling** is a technique used to promote ovulation where we drill small holes into the ovary to reduce cysts and allow drainage.

**Ovarian drilling with laparoscopy** is a technique that may help women who have Polycystic Ovarian Syndrome (PCOS) or Polycystic Ovaries (PCO) to ovulate normally, thus increasing their chances of pregnancy. Ovarian drilling is typically considered after several attempts at ovulation induction using clomid, or an insulin-sensitizing medication, such as metformin. Ovarian drilling cauterizes the stromal theca cells in the ovary. The reduction of this testosterone-producing tissue leads to reduced testosterone levels in the body. Studies have reported that approximately 80% of women who underwent this surgery began ovulating regularly. Post surgery, women who did not regain ovulation, and were previously resistant to clomid citrate, were then more receptive to medical protocols. Pregnancy rates after ovarian drilling are reported at approximately 50%. General anesthesia is administered to the client, and three small incisions are placed in the abdomen. The abdomen is inflated with gas to allow the surgeon to view the ovaries using a laparoscope. The drilling is done by cauterizing different parts of the ovary, and removing the unwanted tissue. The surgeon is able to explore the reproductive system during the laparoscopy, to determine if any additional issues may be present. Ovarian drilling with laparoscopy is an out patient procedure lasting 1-3 hours, plus 1-2 hours of recovery time. Clients can return to work within a week.

**Ovarian wedge resection** is a procedure that is rarely ever used anymore. The belief was that if a part of the ovary was removed, the level of androgens might drop.

## A Chinese Medicine Perspective

Acupuncture has been shown to help relieve symptoms of PCOS by lowering testosterone levels,[cliii] helping to induce ovulation[cliv] and re-establishing menstrual regularity.[clv] When someone walks in with PCOS, we may see any and all of the following symptoms: irregular menstruation, facial hair and acne. Often times the tongue is greasy and swollen with teeth marks, or more of a "geographic tongue" with kidney deficiency, characterized as peeled and shiny on some parts; damp and swollen on other parts. The pulse is almost always slippery and full. The most common Chinese medicine diagnosis with PCOS is damp accumulation with kidney deficiency. In treating PCOS, the goal is to reduce phlegm and resolve waxy capsules around cysts on the ovaries, and regulate the hormonal imbalance causing the cysts. Most often, we use the following points: Sp 9, Sp 6 Zi Gong Xue, along with a back e-stim treatment using UB 23, 52, 32. The herbs: Chong Wei Zi and Zao Jiao Ci help to alleviate damp accumulations in the body along with blood sugar balance.

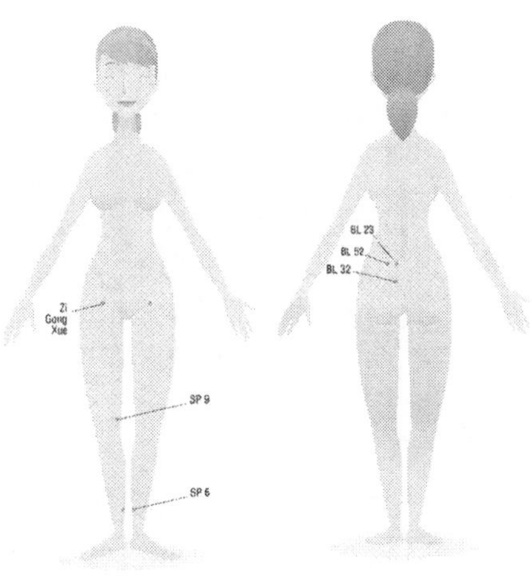


## Diet and Lifestyle Recommendations

Dietary changes also have special significance in helping to treat PCOS. Studies have shown that weight loss, through diet and exercise, as little as 5-10% can be helpful in restoring fertility. A low calorie diet can help balance the menstrual cycle, re-instate ovulation and reduce prevalence of male hormones.[clvi] When obesity is a factor in PCOS, 30% of women have been reported to experience ammenorhea. In women of normal weight only 4.7% did not have a monthly cycle

Regulate blood sugar levels, insulin resistance and excess weight gain by doing the following:

- Partake in a high fiber, low glycemic cleanse like Usana's 5 day RESET program[clvii]

- Eat frequent meals and snacks throughout the day
- Combine a protein and carbohydrate at each meal and snack
- Choose low glycemic foods
- Avoid refined carbohydrates and simple sugars in white breads, pastas, rice, soda, fruit juices, alcohol, high yam consumption
- Avoid caffeine
- Avoid dairy
- Eat abundant cruciferous vegetables (broccoli, cauliflower, brussel sprouts, kale, cabbage, and bok choy) and foods with B vitamins (seaweeds, algaes, legumes, lentils, chickpeas, collard greens, papaya, peas, aparagus, broccoli, strawberries) to metabolize excess estrogen
- Get daily exercise to moderate weight gain (hormones are stored in fat cells)

## Supplementation for PCOS

1. High quality prenatal vitamin/mineral that includes 1000 mcg folic acid
2. Chlorophyll – balances blood sugar levels
3. OPC powder– decreases inflammation and increases circulation, helps to protect body's cells from free radicals damage
4. Fish oil – decrease inflammation, calms reactivity, increase uterine lining quality, overall support for hormonal balance, moderates NK cell activity

5. CoQuinone - increases egg quality by supporting mitochondrial function & energy production

**Yoga Posture for blood sugar balance**

Head to knee stretch (right, then left).

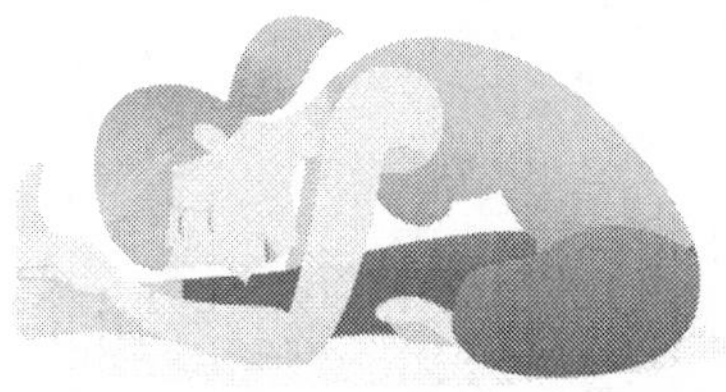

**Massage Recommendations**

Massage can intuitively guide your body back into balance by restoring hormonal balance, in this case, ideally reducing androgens. Because a woman's ovaries need a certain amount of glucose to function, restoring healthy glucose metabolism is essential and can be supported through ATMAM by increasing blood flow to the uterus and ovaries. ATMAM also helps dissolve waxy capsules around cyst, regulate cycles and induce ovulation. Deep work around the sacrum in often indicated and castor oil massage helps to move excess fluid and lymph and reduces inflammation.

## A Mind-Body Perspective

Dr. Northrup believes issues with ovulation can indicate negative feelings about being female, along with stress and repressed pain. She suggests women do the following to realign mind and body:[clviii]

1. Feel negative emotions from childhood fully to release them
2. Re-establish your cyclical flow with life by connecting with the moon and tides
3. Utilize light and nature to heal ovulation-specifically sleeping with the lights on 3 days out of the month

Kristen Magnacca suggests her clients do an exercise to connect with their body and how they might be holding past traumas within. With the help of an Emotional Freedom Technique Practitioner, clients reveal limiting beliefs and associations that may be deeply buried within their cells. Unveiling these thoughts can open the door to deeper healing, helping with the emotional aspect of weight loss.

## Dr. Kiltz Recommends

With PCOS, the most important thing you can do is to adjust your diet and lifestyle. So much of the research is proving that having a healthy BMI (body mass index) can help to restore ovulation.

Daily movement along with a low-glycemic diet can help you to achieve your weight optimization program. Include acupuncture and massage to physically prepare your fertility over three months periods prior to your IVF or natural conception. During those three months, work with a therapist, EFT practitioner, coach or through journaling to uncover repressed emotions from your childhood and embrace your femininity. After three months, have an ultrasound and re-test hormones levels to see where you are at and move forward with the appropriate course of action: natural conception or IVF as the case may be. When embarking on your IVF cycle, we will monitor medications closely to abate the risk of Hyperstimulation Syndrome (OHSS).

## Premature Ovarian Failure (POF)

### By definition…

There is a natural decline in ovarian function as a woman ages. Women are most fertile in their teens and early 20's and fertility declines from then on until they hit menopause. The diagnosis of premature ovarian failure (POF) is given when a woman's egg reserves appear to be declining before the age of 40. At birth, women generally have all the eggs they need to ovulate monthly until approximately age of 50. In the case of POF, something has occurred to alter the supply eggs.

This decline may be the result of the removal of the ovaries, radiation or chemotherapy treatments, hormonal, metabolic or chromosomal issues or autoimmune in nature. POF is believed to effect 1-4% of the population, an estimated 250-000 to 1 million women in the US alone.[clix] The lack of eggs often leads to amenorrhea where women begin to experience symptoms of menopause early.

**Symptoms may include:**

- Amenorrhea (lack of menses) or shortening cycle
- Hot flashes
- Night sweats
- Insomnia
- Mood swings
- Low energy levels
- Low sex drive
- Vaginal dryness
- Pain during sex
- Weakness of the bladder
- High FSH Normal [FSH levels are 10-15 ml U/ml and under; women with POF often have FSH levels above 40 mlU/ml (post-menopausal range)][clx]

**Western Medicine Testing and Treatments**

**Hormone testing and Replacement Therapy** for adrenal, pituitary and thyroid function to locate any deficiencies that might be contributing to the rise in FSH. Estrogen, progesterone and sometimes testosterone are supplemented to restore natural levels. Sometimes birth control is used to reestablish the menstrual cycle. Clomid is often used in an attempt to re-establish ovulation.

Quite often if thyroid and prolactin are normal, not ovulating based on irregular cycles, absent LH rises, clomid is the first line therapy in most western cases. Eastern cases that have shown promise include acupuncture and herbs.

**Genetic testing** for Turner Syndrome and Fragile X syndrome, both impact the X chromosome creating varying levels of ovarian failure.

**Scan for autoimmune conditions and antibodies**: some autoimmune disorders, including Addison's, Hypothyroidism, Systemic Lupus Erythematosus and Type 1 Diabetes have been associated with the early onset of menopause. In unnamed forms of autoimmunity antibodies may attack the cells producing reproductive hormones, causing ovarian failure.

**History of specific illnesses and STD's** make premature ovarian failure more likely including inflammatory conditions like sarcoidosis, mumps, epilepsy and tuberculosis.

**Egg preservation**: where POF is an expected outcome of cancer radiation treatment, embryo cryopreservation is the most for freezing fertilized eggs for later IVF treatments. Other potential treatments include freezing unfertilized eggs and removing part of the ovary to be re-implanted after cancer treatments. Hormone therapy during chemotherapy is also being tested to understand the potential impact of preserving the ovaries.

**IVF with donor eggs** is an often recommended and a very viable option for those with POF.

**A Chinese Medicine Perspective**

When a client comes in with the diagnosis of POF, we work with the symptoms presented to us including: high FSH, poor ovarian response in stimulation, and/or irregular or absent period. We usually see a tongue that is shiny and red with no coating and a deep and weak kidney pulse. From an Eastern standpoint, the equivalent diagnosis is kidney essence or yin deficiency, and we look for signs of low back or knee pain, prematurely grey hair, vaginal dryness, scanty cervical mucus, dark eye circles, hot flashes and fear. With a desire to bring back regular menses and ovulation and re-establish communication along the HPO axis with the conception and governing meridians to connect the heart and uterus, our treatment strategy is all about restoring blood flow to the uterus and ovaries and nourishing blood and estrogen. Two common treatments use acupuncture points: Kidney 3, 6, Spleen 6 and Zi Gong Shui around ovaries and e-stim back treatments using UB 23, 52, 32 (contra-indicated after ovulation, and if you think you might be pregnant). The herbal formulas six flavors, women's precious help to re-establish menses by transformation stasis to invigorate blood flow.

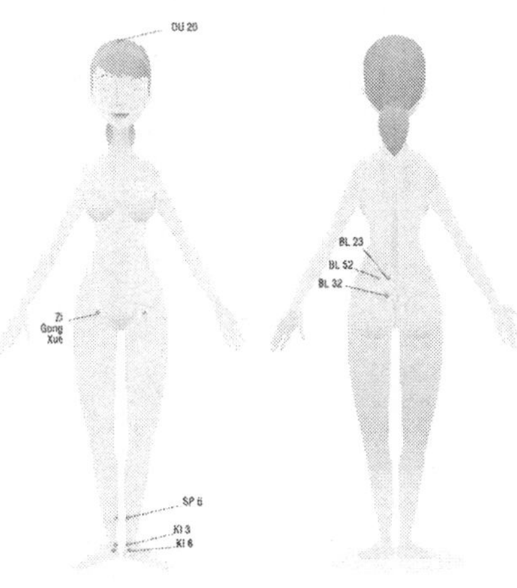


**Study from Fertile Soul Database: Acupuncture can stimulate ovulation without risk[clxi]**

Human menopausal gonadotropin (HMG) and human chorionic gonadotropin (HCG) are often used in the artificial induction of ovulation. With these two hormones, the ovulatory rate was about 70%-90%, but the incidence of ovarian hyperstimulation syndrome (OHSS) might be 10%-15.4% and even life threatening in severe cases. At present, there are no satisfactory measures for the prevention and remission of OHSS It is considered that when OHSS occurs, stopping injection of HCG is the effective way to avoid severe OHSS. However, stopping HCG not only discontinues the ovulation, but also causes the loss of the already developed follicles. Our clinical practice demonstrated that acupuncture is effective in ovulation induction (without hormone injections) and also in the remission of OHSS induced by injected HMG.

**Diet and Lifestyle Recommendations**

The key component of re-establishing healthy ovulation patterns is to build yin in your system to nourish blood and fertility. Apart from the regular fertility guidelines, we recommend:

- Foods to cool and build reserves: apple, asparagus, bananas, barley, bean sprouts, beets, blackberry, bulgur, cheese, chlorella, chickpeas, clam, crab, cuttlefish, duck, eggplant, eggs, honey, grapes, kidney bean, jellyfish, lemon, malt, mango, melon, milk, mulberry, organ meats, oyster, pea, pear, pineapples, pomegranate, pork, rabbit, raspberries, rice, seaweed, shellfish, spirulina, string bean, tofu, tomato, watermelon, and yam.
- Avoid hot and spicy foods, which might

exacerbate heat symptoms

- Replace caffeinated beverages with any of the vast array of healing teas: chamomile (calming), ginger (warming, supportive of digestion), red clover (believed to enhance fertility) and peppermint (cooling).
- Avoid alcohol, tobacco and unnecessary medications.
- Build essence with chlorophyll rich foods: dark leafy greens, seaweed, and algae's: wheat grass.
- ALWAYS eat organic to avoid excess estrogens, which will imbalance the system.
- At least one activity that brings you peace and calm each day with a deep restful period
- Replenishing activities like yoga and qi gong that connect the breath with movement; swimming is also wonderfully restorative (especially in salt water).

## Supplementation to Treat High FSH and Egg Quality

1. High quality prenatal vitamin/mineral that includes 1000 mcg folic acid
2. CoQuinone – increases egg quality by supporting mitochondrial function & energy production
3. Wheat Grass – improves egg quality by lowering FSH levels
4. Royal Jelly – improves egg quality by adding essential nutrients to the cells

5. Fish oil – decrease inflammation, calms reactivity, increase uterine lining quality, overall support for hormonal balance, moderates NK cell activity

**Yoga Posture for Premature Ovarian Failure**

Forward bends support deep relaxation of the nervous system.

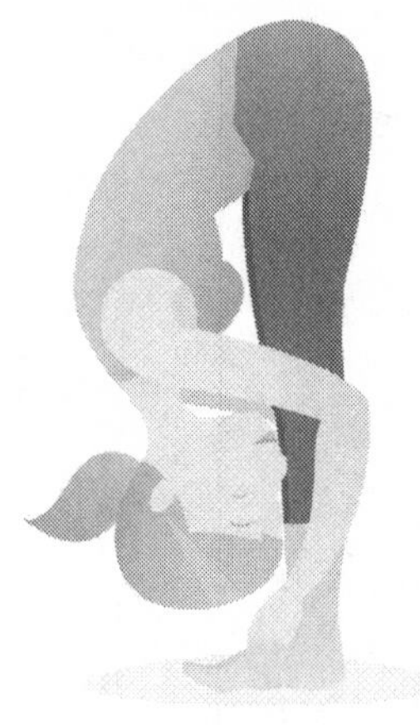

**Massage Recommendations**

Ovulation is based on hemodynamic, the flow of blood through the body. If blood flow is not adequate, ovulation patterns are affected. Proper positioning of the uterus and ovaries through ATMAM is essential for supporting blood flow and transport of hormones necessary for the ovulatory process. The femoral massage (see luteal phase defect section) is a specific technique that localizes nourishing blood flow to the reproductive organs, but briefly cuts off blood flow by pressing on the femoral artery, and subsequently releasing it, to release a gush of blood. Beyond being beneficial directly for reproductive function, massage has been shown to have incredible results on reducing stress. In a study published in the International Journal of Neurosciences (2004), researchers studied the effect of moderate, light or vibratory massage on stress levels by studying brain waves and heartbeat. All three groups reported decreased stress and anxiety, the largest drop being in the moderate pressure group.[clxii]

## A Mind-Body Perspective

Reducing stress levels can feel like it's "easier said than done" in this busy world. And yet, each day we have the opportunity to choose to put ourselves first and introduce relaxation and sanity back into our lives. Taking an inventory of activities that are causing us stress or where fear is arising can be helpful in recreating patterns that support our highest good. Often just confronting our fear allows them to slip away. Physiologically, the relaxation response developed by Benson to combat the fight flight response is one of the most profound and simple acts to return our bodies to balance. Taking moments to tense all of our body parts and release them can flood our body with fresh oxygen and reset our pattern. Deep breath work partnered with meditation is also helpful and even some moments in between meetings can really make a difference. Focus on your second chakra, your seat of creativity and power and visualize the color orange as you meditate to activate your fertile energies. Keeping a gratitude list that you can add to each day also helps to reestablish the natural outward flow of the heart in flooding the body with positive sentiments and vibrations.

**Dr. Kiltz Recommends**

I believe that premature ovarian is best treated using a combination of modalities. Western medicine uses testing along with hormone therapy, and generally recommends supplementing with the hormones the body is lacking. It may also make sense to think ahead and consider preserving your eggs. What is important is that before you move forward with a donor cycle, give yourself time to sit with it. Take the time you need to make the decision that is right for you, before rushing into anything. Finding your intuition in this process is the gift of learning to slow down and hear your inner voice. As more and more research is being conducted into the fight flight response and its ability to impact the HPO axis, it is important to look at your life and ask yourself where you could draw in relaxation each day. Meditate, breathe and read quietly. Your daily thoughts and activities directly influence your physiology. Setting aside time each day for seated meditation with one hand on your belly (2nd chakra) and one hand on your heart has the potential to regenerate your entire system.

## Structural Blockages

**By definition…**

When the path from a woman's ovaries to the uterus is not cleared, conception becomes difficult and sometimes impossible through natural conception. Structural blockages can be the result of several factors, including pelvic inflammatory disease (PID) from sexually transmitted diseases like chlamydia or gonorrhea, IUD's commonly leading to fallopian tube obstructions and uterine or pelvic adhesions from surgical procedures or scarring from infections, history of ectopic pregnancy, endometriosis or a ruptured appendix. In one particular type of blockage, a hydrosalpinx, the blockage causes the tube to fill with fluid or pus (pyrosalpinx), blocking the egg and sperm, preventing fertilization and implantation.

**Symptoms and Indicators:**

- Pelvic pain
- History of Ectopic pregnancy (pelvic pain, low lingering HCG levels, no intrauterine gestational sac, spotting, discharge)

- Spotting during pregnancy
- Irregular cycle
- Vaginal discharge
- Restricted movement

**Western Medicine Testing and Treatment**

**Hysterosalpingogram (HSG):** in this specialized procedure, dye is inserted through the cervix. An x-ray of the pelvis is taken to observe whether the dye moves easily through the uterus and the fallopian tubes. With this test, there is a 15% chance of a false positive. The fallopian tubes are sometimes reactive to the dye and can go into spasms most often at the point where the tube and uterus meet. If this happens, your Reproductive Endocrinologist would most likely repeat the test.

**Regular or Trans-vaginal Ultrasound** is used as a diagnostic tool to look for any irregularities in the pelvic cavity, an ultrasound is unable to see scar tissue, which has the appearance of crushed cellophane, but may show a dilated fallopian tube as the result of an infection or potentially indicating a hydrosalpinx.

**Hysteroscopy:** in this procedure a thin camera is inserted through the cervix to examine the uterus, providing helpful diagnostic information.

**Laparoscopic surgery** can sometimes remove adhesions and blockages, improving the chances of a healthy pregnancy (20-40% chance of conceiving if tube is otherwise healthy). If the scarring is minor, this surgery may be helpful, but in the case of a hydrosalpinx or major scarring between the ovary and tube, surgery is not a good option and IVF treatment may be indicated. Surgeons may even remove the unhealthy portion of the fallopian tube and re-attach it using laser surgery.

**Pressure lavage under ultrasound guidance (PLUG)** is a procedure used to clear out mild scarring in the uterus. Using a transvaginal sonohysterography, an ultrasound that tracks the infusion of saline into the uterus aiding in the breaking up of scar tissue.

A **Chlamydia** antibody test may be ordered to show any history of sexually transmitted disease that may have contributed to the structural blockage.

**IVF** is the best option where both tubes are blocked and surgery is not a viable option, even more so when there is male factor.

**Methotrexate:** when ectopic pregnancy is suspected, methotrexate is the best course of action to avoid full surgery and the possibility of scar tissue. Methotrexate is a drug used in the treatment of some cancers and autoimmune conditions that stops the replication of cells. In the case of ectopic pregnancy that is not too far advanced, it may be used to end the pregnancy, allowing it to reabsorb into the body without invasive treatment.

**A Chinese Medicine Perspective**

With structural blockages and pelvic adhesions, there is usually no physical manifestation to be seen through Chinese medicine pulse or tongue diagnosis. However, along with the Western diagnosis of tubal blockages or pelvic adhesions, the acupuncturist's most common diagnosis will be obstruction of Qi and blood or phlegm and or damp heat, which will guide the treatment strategy.

One of the most common channels to use in treating excess discharge is through the Dai Mai, or Girdle meridian which is one of the extraordinary meridians that allows excesses from all the organs to be discharged.[clxiii] Acupuncture is also helpful in treating underlying conditions including emotional distress, while physical manipulation through Maya Abdominal Massage or the Wurn technique is best for alleviating mechanical blockages.

Some of the herbs used to unblock fallopian tubes include: milk thistle, horsetail, burdock, crampbark, pine tree bark and vitex. According to a 1995 Chinese study, herbs were used to treat pelvic inflammatory disease that can lead to mechanical blockages. For 20-60 days, 148 women received treatment with a combination of Xiao Yal San Jia

Wei (Rambling Powder with Added Flavors) and Kang Fu Xiao Yan Shuan (Healthy Woman Disperse Inflammation Suppository) with a 97% cure rate in the removal of adhesions and the restoration uterus and fallopian tubes to a healthy state.[clxiv]

**Diet and Lifestyle Recommendations**

Nutrition can help to restore the free flow of energy and nutrients to every area of the body.

- When there are blockages and stagnations cook with spices like basil, caraway, cardamom, cayenne, chive, clove, coriander, dill seed, garlic, marjoram, mustard leaf, orange peel, peppermint, rosemary, spearmint, star anise, tangerine peel, thyme and turmeric.
- To address phlegm and dampness avoid the following damp foods: cow's milk products, pork, roasted peanuts, fruit juices, wheat, yeast, breads, alcohol, bananas, sugar, sweeteners and saturated fats.
- The following foods can help to alleviate phlegm: almonds, apple peel, clam, garlic, grapefruit, kelp, lemon peel, licorice, marjoram, button mushrooms, mustard leaf, mustard seed, olive, onion, orange peel, pear, black pepper, white pepper, peppermint, persimmon, plantain, radish, seaweed, shitake mushroom, shrimp, tea,

thyme, walnuts.

- Apart from eliminating cow dairy, wheat and sugar can all exacerbate inflammation and trying goat dairy, gluten free products and low-glycemic sweeteners is a good idea. Eating an omega rich diet also helps to reduce inflammation: salmon, mackeral, tuna, flaxseed oil, evening primrose oil, pumpkin seed oil, black currant oil, linseed oil
- Gentle movements like Qi Gong and yoga can also encourage the free flow of energy through the meridians and can be a meditative technique to help relax the system.

**Supplementation for Structural Blockages**

1. High quality prenatal vitamin/mineral that includes 1000 mcg folic acid
2. Fish oil (4000 mg/day) - decrease inflammation, calms reactivity, increase uterine lining quality, overall support for hormonal balance, moderates NK cell activity
3. OPC powder– decreases inflammation and increases circulation, helps to protect body's cells from free radicals damage
4. Nattokanise – helps break up adhesions and prevent clotting

## Massage Recommendations

Castor oil massage is deeply soothing and helpful in alleviate pain, increase circulation and dislodge tubal blockages and pelvic adhesions. Massage helps break up scar tissue and realigns the organs to create structural balance that promotes healthy blood flow. The founder of the Arvigo Technique of Maya Abdominal Massage considered hemodynamics, the study of the forces involved in the obstruction of blood flow, in the application of ATMAM. She believes that miracles happen when blood flow returns and stagnancy is released. External and internal techniques can both be used to dislodge blockages in the fallopian tubes and break up pelvic adhesions. Preliminary research on the Wurn Technique, developed by Clear Passages, has also revealed a notable reversal in 75% of cases that showed tubal blockages.[clxv] Craniosacral is also a wonderful technique for re-aligning the pelvis and the spine to support fallopian tube health.[clxvi] Massage on the abdominal area is to be done prior to ovulation and avoided during menstruation.

## Yoga Posture: To promote free flow of energy in the pelvis

Cat Cow Stretch helps to align the spine, support blood flow and proper nerve function, promoting free flowing energy and movement internally and externally.

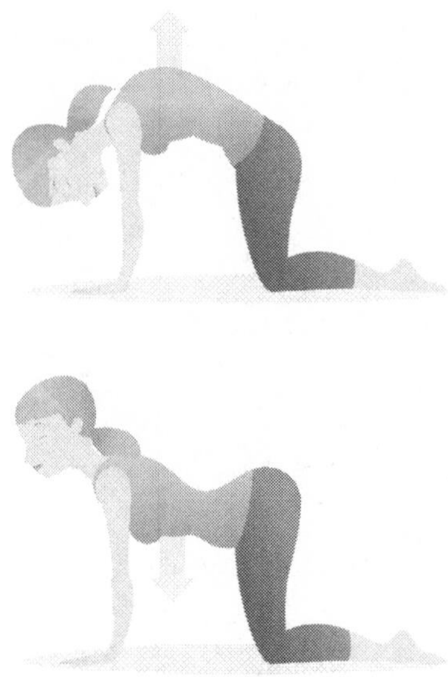

## A Mind-Body Perspective

Mechanical blockages may indicate an overall block in your energy flow. 15% of HSG tests are false positives for blockages because fear and anxiety can actually create spasms in the fallopian tubes.

"When I went through the process, I knew in my heart I hadn't lost my tubal function. Yet, when the test went horribly wrong, and reported I had no tubal function, the rational part of my husband and doctor's mind took over, dismissing the idea that there was any mistake. I trusted my intuition, refusing to look at this test as a black and white situation and set myself a date in the future to become pregnant naturally before moving

forward with IVF. One day prior to my date I conceived. The mind is a powerful ally when we focus on the possibility. Positive affirmation like 'I am in my flow' always helped me to keep my sights on my intention."
— Kristen Magnacca

**Dr. Kiltz Recommends**

Structural blockages account for approximately 50% of all infertility cases. While some can be reversed with surgeries and even a routine HSG scan where the dye removes the block, we are lucky to have IVF as an option. I feel strongly that clients should be advised of the limitations of all tests and always encourage holding the intention of healing in your mind as you go forward always. I think it is really important that clients be aware of all the options available to them. There is great research about massage techniques, and ultimately, if a couple decides to pursue IVF, they will have improved the quality of their eggs by increasing blood flow both through massage, acupuncture and dietary techniques.

**Unexplained Infertility**
**By definition…**

Unexplained fertility is the diagnosis given when there is no apparent medical reason as to why a couple is not conceiving. About 10% of couples diagnosed with infertility will have unexplained infertility. This is perhaps one of the most frustrating diagnoses for a woman, because there is no known factor for why she is not becoming pregnant. It is suspected that stress may play a large factor in unexplained fertility and using an integrative approach to balancing the body with diet, exercise, massage, meditation, acupuncture helps to reestablish healthy reproductive function. If after all the following tests are run, and nothing shows up, a diagnosis of unexplained fertility is given, because there is no known medical reason the couple is not conceiving.

**Western Medicine Tests and Treatments**

1. Verify normal ovulation patterns
2. HSG test to ensure your fallopian tubes are open and healthy
3. Rule out pelvic adhesions
4. Determine that no endometriosis is present
5. Sperm health panel for partner
6. A postcoital test to evaluate the interaction between the sperm and cervical mucous

**A Chinese Medicine Perspective**

In Chinese medicine there is always a diagnosis it is never unexplained because everyone has an underlying pattern of imbalance that can be brought into greater balance. The key is to find energetic imbalance and treat it accordingly. Usually, clients with the diagnosis of unexplained fertility present with noticeable high stress levels shown in their wiry, tight pulse and moderate to dark tongue. The most common Chinese medicine diagnosis is Liver Qi stagnation and lack of blood flow to the reproductive system. The treatment strategy is reduce fight or flight by moderating the cortisol levels in the adrenals and reestablishing healthy nervous system function using a combination of points including LI4, Liv 3 and Yin tang or, alternatively, e-stim on UB 23, 52, 32, both before ovulation. A favorite herbal remedy to reduce stress is Xiao Yao San, named free and easy wanderer because it helps take away the angst and allows normally over-stressed people to float through their day. A 2004 study measured the effectiveness of treating unexplained infertility through Chinese Medicine finding over half the women became pregnant within a six month period.[clxvii]

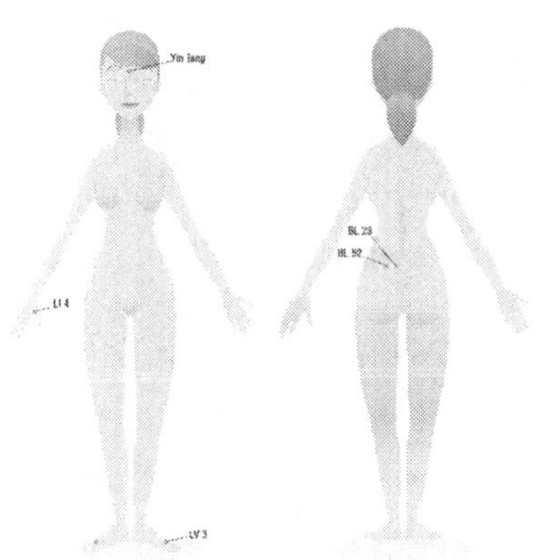

## Diet and Lifestyle Recommendations

In line with the Chinese medicine diagnosis of Liver Qi stagnation, steps can be taken nutritionally to calm the system by removing any agitants from the diet, most notably caffeine, alcohol, unnecessary prescription drugs and sugar. Because the proper distribution of nutrients from the digestive system directly impacts the liver's ability to process stress and the hormones, it is a good idea to use the basic fertility diet guidelines by replacing wheat and refined carbohydrates along with dairy. Stabilizing blood sugar levels by eating small frequent meals and snacks throughout the day can also go along way to stabilizing mood. Going to sleep before 11pm each night to ensure the liver and gallbladder times for regeneration is optimized, along with replenishing exercise and adequate relaxation, will ensure we are combating the stress response with the relaxation response.

## Supplementation for Unexplained Infertility

1. High quality prenatal vitamin/mineral that includes 1000 mcg folic acid
2. OPC powder– decreases inflammation and increases circulation, helps to protect body's cells from free radicals damage
3. Fish oil – decrease inflammation, overall support for hormonal balance

## Yoga Posture for Unexplained Fertility

Savasana: lie on your back with your palms facing up. Practice the relaxation response by tightening all of your muscles, beginning with the feet all the way to the top of your head. Hold for 30 seconds and release, laying in silence for an additional 5-10 minutes. This simple but profound act relaxes the nervous system and is believed to be the equivalent of a full night's rest.

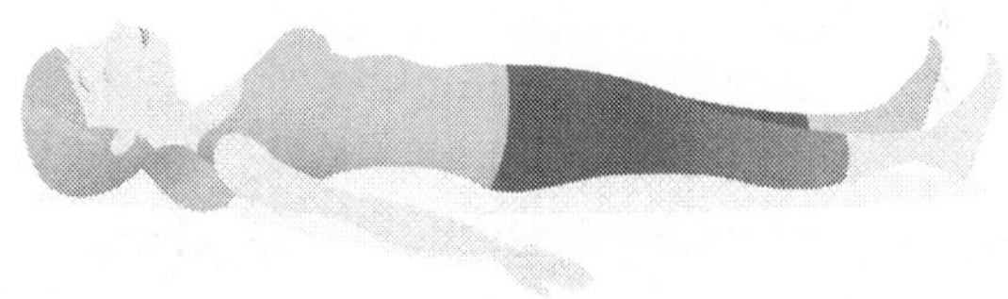

## Massage Recommendations

Massage for stress reduction is key. Many of the women that we see at CNY Fertility & Healing Arts who have been diagnosed with unexplained infertility are real go-getters in their day-to-day life; stress plays a big part of their diagnosis. Long-term exposure to elevated cortisol levels disturbs hormone balance and reproductive health. In a study published in the International Journal of Neurosciences (2004), researchers studied the effect of moderate, light or vibratory massage on stress levels, by studying brain waves and heartbeat. All three groups reported decreased stress and anxiety, the largest drop being in the moderate pressure group.[clxviii] Massage can help by rebalancing the yin and yang element and reconnecting the women with her body and needs. It can also help the body to detox, relax and learn self-awareness. Supporting proper pelvic alignment and increasing blood flow to the uterus and ovaries can only be beneficial; it provides women with physical and emotional benefits.

## A Mind-Body Perspective

Not knowing can be the hardest part. At least when we have a specific diagnosis, we feel more in control of the outcome. Uncertainty can send us into a tailspin but it is more important than ever to create opportunities to induce the relaxation response through breath work, positive affirmation, soothing music and activities that bring you pleasure. As we know the connection between the heart and uterus is paramount with fertility and stress literally creates a kink in our system, holding the breath and blood flow in the chest. Practicing the microcosmic breath, deep belly breathing, for even a few moments each day can help to reset these patterns. By placing one hand on the heart and one hand on the uterus, you are energetically encouraging the conception meridian to open, supporting reproductive function. You might also place your palms on your lower back on each side of your spine. The reproductive organs are the paired organs of the kidneys and you can literally provide nourishment with the healing touch of your own hands.

**Dr. Kiltz Recommends**

Never do I see clients as frustrated as when they receive the diagnosis of unexplained infertility. However, these days when you consider the research on the impact of stress, unexplained infertility open many doors for rebalancing with natural healing techniques and a true reassessment of our habitual patterns that may be contributing to the temporary block in our fertility. Taking out stimulants in your diet, getting adequate rest and incorporating activities that bring you peace and joy is paramount. Acupuncture and massage are proven techniques that change the flow of your energy and elicit the relaxation response. Last but not least, practice deep belly breathing often, sooner or later it will become a habit.

# Acknowledgements

Nothing happens by itself, it all takes energy from the Creator, and that I acknowledge first and foremost. To all of those that have guided me in my life: my teachers, professors, my family, friends, coworkers and clients, and most of all to those that have contributed to this book with their thoughts and their knowledge.

To Kathryn Flynn and her persistence in bringing together the people and their energy so that together we can share different ways that all of us can find the secret of life, which is really not a secret. It is through knowledge that we may find it, in front of us, within us, and around all of us. Kathryn has helped bring this knowledge together in one place.

I thank Justine Taylor, Erin McCollough, Heather Smith, Kristen Magnacca, Lisa Stack, Jessie Briel, April, Coburn Design and many others that are not written down here for their contributions to the content within. This knowledge has been written down many times before, by many different people, I am not the first. In this book, we are sharing it in a way that I believe is different, and it is our intent to have our version speak to you. We must recognize that this power is truly within all of us.

Thank you to all of you whom, at this very

moment, are taking the time to read the pages of this book and are going through struggles, (I like to call them gifts), on this journey of learning in life. We must learn to experience our true inner flow in order to glow in life. This is the secret, the fertile secret.

Love,

Dr. Rob

# Fertile Secret Contributors

## Assisted Reproductive Medicine

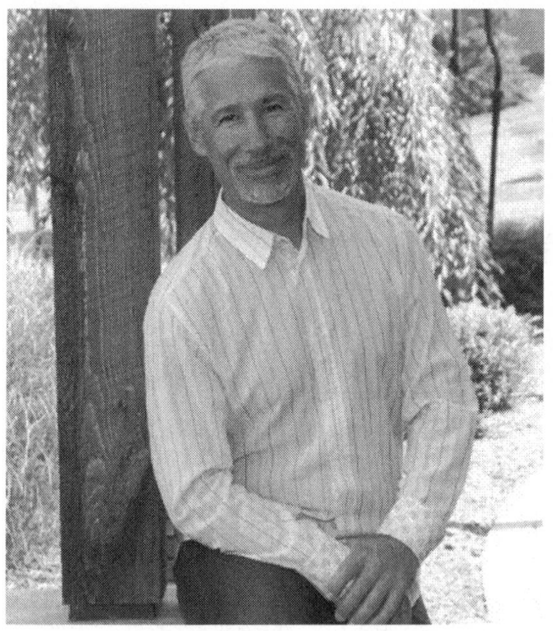

*Robert J. Kiltz, MD FACOG Founder/Director CNY Fertility and Healing Arts*

Dr. Robert Kiltz, MD, is founder and director of Central New York's first successful IVF center, CNY Fertility Center, where he focuses on his passion of combining spiritual practices with ART (Assisted Reproductive Technologies).

In addition to his work at CNY Fertility Center, he is also the Owner / Director of CNY Healing Arts Center, an accomplished artist, and a motivational speaker. His practice embraces both the newest Western technologies and the oldest Eastern philosophies. It is a formula that has been successful for both his patients and himself.

His life's work is to help others reach their spiritual goals, achieve happiness and success, and live spectacular lives by creating balance and wellness within oneself. Life is about experience, love, challenge, and understanding. When we have the tools to accept these things into our lives, we create an abundance of joy around us.

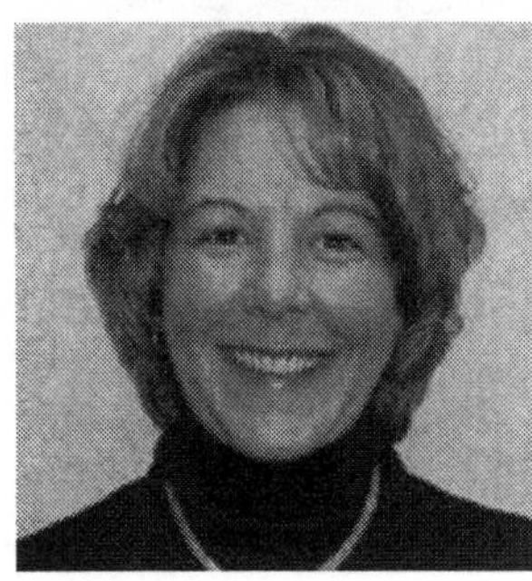

*Justine Taylor, RN, BSN Nurse Manager and IVF Coordinator*

Justine coordinates the IVF cycles in our Latham

office of CNY Fertility. She monitors patient stimulation cycles with ultrasound. She performs blood draws, patient education and intrauterine inseminations. She also oversees the daily operation of the Latham office and its staff. She is a graduate of Samaritan Hospital School of Nursing in Troy, NY and The State University of New York at Utica/Rome in Utica, New York. She has worked in women's health for 21 years, specializing in Reproductive Medicine since 1994.

## Chinese Medicine

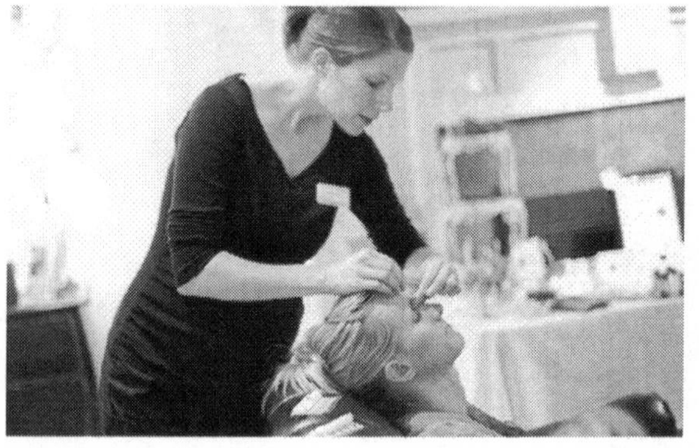

*Heather Smith, L.Ac.*

Heather is a NY State Licensed Acupuncturist as well as a Chinese Herbalist. She received her Masters Degree in Acupuncture from the American College of Acupuncture and Oriental Medicine in Houston, TX. Additionally, Heather received her

Bachelors of Science in Health Science with a concentration in wellness and health promotion. The primary focus in Heather's Chinese Medical Practice is fertility. Her experience in treating issues related to fertility began while working with Dr. Randine Lewis, distinguished Acupuncturist and Author of The Infertility Cure. After years of learning the art of healing from Dr. Lewis, Heather has a comprehensive knowledge of treating various conditions related to fertility and hormonal response. Although fertility is her main focus, Heather's education and clinical training give her the experience necessary to treat a variety of conditions, including but not limited to, depression, menopause, immune issues, anxiety, stress and insomnia.

## CNY Client Experience

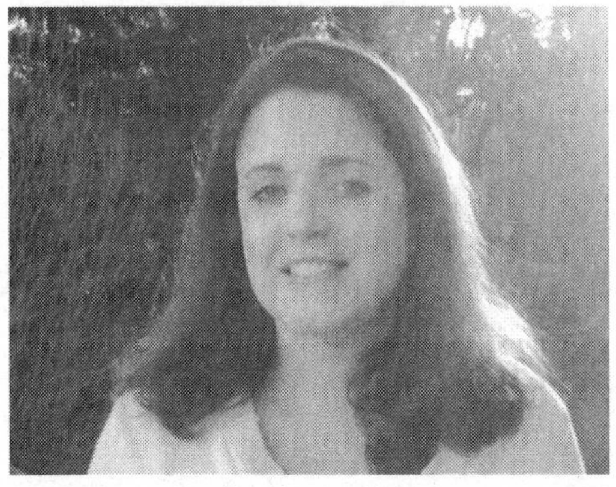

April, CNY Fertility Client and Blogger

April is a CNY Fertility Center patient and has been on her journey to fertility for approximately two and a half years. April shares candid stories and a unique perspective on the fertility challenges many women and couples face. April became pregnant in 2011 and delivered a healthy baby in 2012. She is one of our many Success Stories!

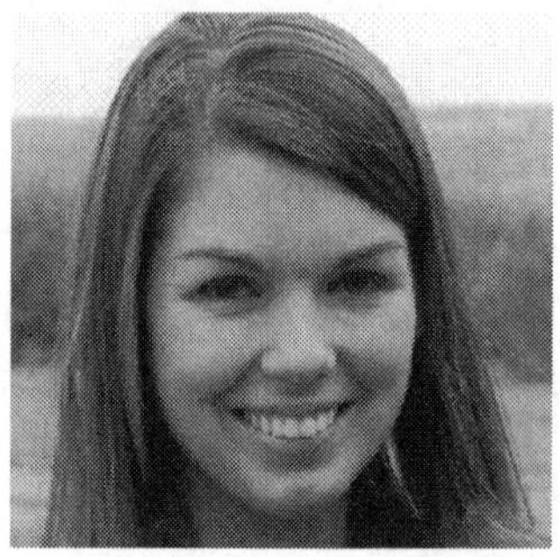

*Lisa Stack, Support Coordinator*

Lisa is the support coordinator at CNY Fertility Center and assists our clients on their journey toward fertility by offering help and suggestions to work through the daily challenges they encounter. Please feel free to contact her for any of your support questions or needs.

## Massage

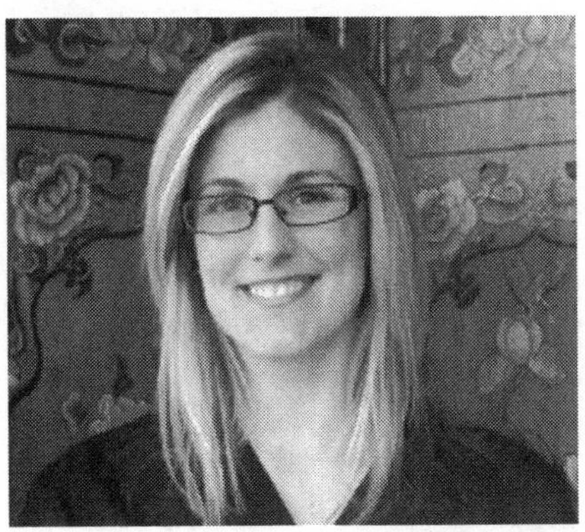

*Erin McCollough LMT, RYT*

Erin uses her twelve years experience of practicing complementary medicine to help nurture and support the reproductive health of women. Erin attended both Penn State University and Syracuse University to obtain a Bachelors of Science. While attending Syracuse University, Erin enrolled in a yoga class. That choice has forever changed her life. Since then, she obtained a degree from the Onondaga School of Therapeutic Massage and is both a NYS licensed massage therapist as well as a nationally certified massage therapist through the NCBTMB. In addition, Erin completed the Essential Yoga Teacher Training, is a Registered Yoga Teacher through the Yoga Alliance, and has completed both professional training in The Arvigo Techniques of Maya Abdominal Therapy (ATMAT) and advanced ATMAT for fertility and pregnancy (www.arvigomassage.com). Her own journey into motherhood is her inspiration for assisting women to obtain optimal fertility and reproductive health.

## Mind-Body

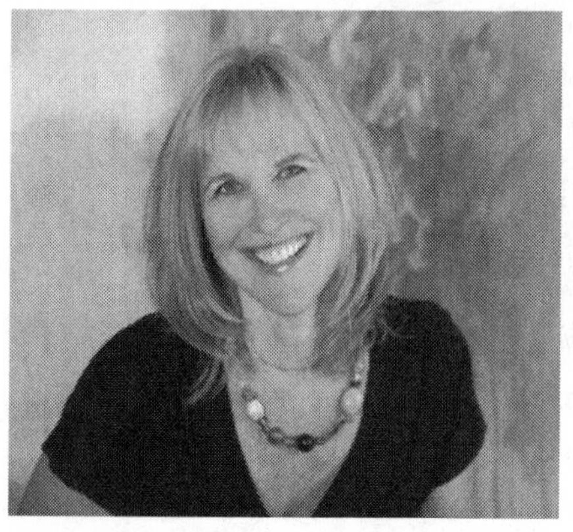

*Kristen Magnacca is the author of Girlfriend To Girlfriend: A Fertility Companion and Love & Infertility: Survival Strategies for Balancing Infertility, Marriage and Life and the recipient of RESOLVE'S 2009 Hope Award for Best Book!*

Kristen Magnacca has served as an expert on the emotional aspects of infertility, testifying before the US Senate in the spring of 2000 about the importance of government funding for fertility research and holistic treatment. She has been highlighted in national publications and broadcast media including NBC's The Today Show, Woman's World magazine, PBS' Health Week and The Boston Globe. She is also a past board member and volunteer of RESOLVE of the Bay State and works with fertility clinics and fertility providers to help them to enhance and improve the fertility patient's experience. Kristen lives with her husband, Mark, and their children, Grace and Cole, in East Sandwich, Massachusetts.

## Diet and Lifestyle

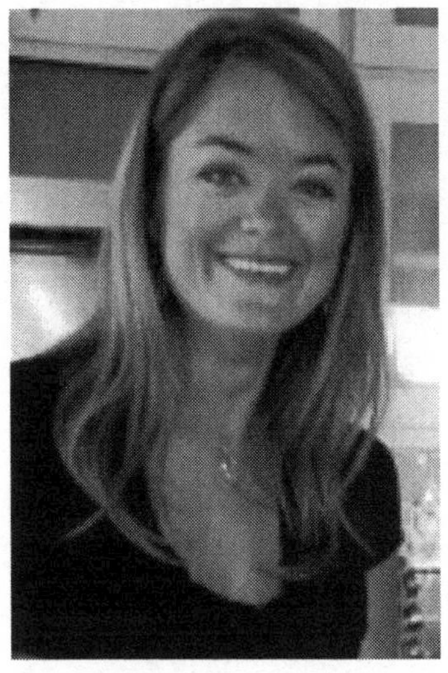

*Kathryn Simmons Flynn, B. Ed, is the author of Cooking for Fertility: Foods to Nourish Your Fertile Soul, Healing with Whole Foods, The Infertility Cure* and *The Way of the Fertile Soul.*

Kathryn Simmons Flynn studied with Paul Pitchford, author of Healing with Whole Foods, and has worked extensively with Dr. Randine Lewis, author of The Infertility Cure and The Way of the Fertile Soul, to develop The Fertile Soul's integrative nutrition program for reproductive health (www.thefertilesoul.com). She provides individual nutritional counseling to men and women worldwide, with the intention of enhancing reproductive capacity naturally through a holistic approach that includes lifestyle changes, relaxation techniques, exercise and healing foods. Kathryn is the founder of Fertile Foods, a website intended to educate men and women about food and lifestyle habits to support a healthy pregnancy (www.fertilefoods.com).

# Notes

---

[i] *Office on Women's Health: Frequently asked questions* (2009, June 1). Retrieved February 12, 2010, from http://www.womenshealth.gov/faq/infertility.cfm

[ii] *Fertility: The Mind/Body Connection: An Overview* (2009, August 27). Retrieved February 12, 2010, from http://www.infertilitymindbody.com

[iii] Northrup, M.D., D. (2009, August 27). *Enhancing Fertility: A Mind/Body Perspective.* Retrieved February 12, 2010, from http://www.drnorthrup.com/womenshealth/healthcenter/topic_details.php?topic_id=124

[iv] *Fertility: The Mind/Body Connection: An Overview* (2009, August 27). Retrieved February 12, 2010, from http://www.infertilitymindbody.com

[v] Schell, FJ., Allolio, B., Schonecke, OW. (1994) Physiological and psychological effects of Hatha yoga exercise in healthy women. Int. J. Psychosom. 41: 46-52.

[vi] Mate , G. (2003). *When the Body Says No: Understanding the Stress-Disease Connection.* Vancouver: John Wiley & Sons, Inc. 61.

[vii] Benson, H. The Relaxation Response. New York: William Morrow 1975

---

[viii] Benson, H. The Relaxation Response (1975). Retrieved February 12, 2010, from http://relaxationresponse.org/steps/

[ix] *Canadian Federation for Sexual Health Female Reproductive Anatomy* (2008, June 28). Retrieved February 12, 2010, from http://www.cfsh.ca/Your_Sexual_Health/Anatomy/Female_Reproductive_Anatomy.aspx

[x] Kern, D. (2009, August 28). Retrieved February 12, 2010, from http://drdebkern.com/resources/dr-debs-handouts/

[xi] Lewis, R. (2005, June 1). *High FSH: Acupuncture and Herbal Therapy for Enhancing Egg Quality* . Retrieved February 12, 2010, from http://www.resolve.org/site/PageServer?pagename=cop_ch_20050601

[xii] Lipton, Ph.D. , B. H. (2004). *Eastern Medicine and Western Science: The Grand Convergence* . Retrieved February 12, 2010, from http://www.tcmabc.org/news/articles/eastern-medicine-western-science.php

[xiii] Emoto, M. (2004). *The Hidden Messages in Water* . Oregon: Beyond Words Publishing.

[xiv] Lewis, R. (2006). *Fertility Enhancing DVD Lecture Series, Session A: Nourishing Your Fertile Soul: Enhancing the Reproductive Response* . Asheville: The Fertile Soul.

---

[xv] Tamura et al, H. (2006). Melatonin and the ovary: physiological and pathophysiological implications. *Fertility and Sterility*, *92*(1), 328-343. Retrieved February 12, 2010, from http://www.ncbi.nlm.nih.gov/pubmed/18804205?itool=EntrezSystem2.PEntrez.Pubmed.Pubmed_ResultsPanel.Pubmed_RVDocSum&ordinalpos=1

[xvi] Hagelin, J. S., Rainforth, M. V., C. Cavanaugh, K. L., Alexander, C. N., Shatkin, S. F., Davies, J. L., Hughes, Anne O., Ross, Emanuel, Orme-Johnson, David W. et al. Effects of Group Practice of the Transcendental Meditation Program on Preventing Violent Crime in Washington, D.C.: Results of the National Demonstration Project. , *93*(June), 153-201. Retrieved February 12, 2010, from http://www.alltm.org/pages/crime-arrested.html

[xvii] Hagelin, J. S. (1999, June 1). *Transcendental Meditation Experiment Arrests Crime Study Shows Dramatic Drop in Violent Crime During D.C. Project* . Retrieved February 12, 2010, from http://www.alltm.org/pages/crime-arrested.html

[xviii] Doidge, N. (2007). *The Brain that Changes Itself, Stories of Personal Triumph from the Frontiers of Brain Science*. England: Penguin Books, 203-204

[xix] Mate , G. (2003). *When the Body Says No: Understanding the Stress-Disease Connection*. Vancouver: John Wiley & Sons, Inc., 239

---

[xx] Bolton Taylor, J. (2008, February). *My Stroke of Insight*. Retrieved February 12, 2010, from http://www.ted.com/index.php/talks/jill_bolte_taylor_s_powerful_stroke_of_insight.html

[xxi] Dale, C. (2009). *The Subtle Body An Encyclopedia of Your Energetic Anatomy*. Boulder : Sounds True. , 27

[xxii] Kern, D. (2009, August 28). *Brave Grace.* Retrieved February 12, 2010, from http://drdebkern.com/speaking/keynote-topics/

[xxiii] Dale, C. (2009). *The Subtle Body An Encyclopedia of Your Energetic Anatomy*. Boulder : Sounds True. , 45.

[xxiv] Amen, D. G. (1998). *Change Your Brain Change Your Life, The Breakthrough Program for Conquering Anxiety, Depression, Obsessiveness, Anger and Impulsiveness*. New York: Three Rivers Press., 57

[xxv] *Nuclear Age Peace Foundation* (1998). Retrieved February 12, 2010, from http://www.wagingpeace.org/menu/issues/peace-&-war/start/peace-quotes/

[xxvi] Summary Of Secret Teachings (2007). Retrieved February 12, 2010, from http://thesecret.tv/top-secret-summary-of-teachings.html

---

[xxvii] The Secret: Trailer (2007). Retrieved February 12, 2010, from http://thesecret.tv/top-secret-summary-of-teachings.htmlhttp://thesecret.tv/movie/trailer.html

[xxviii] The Work of Byron Katie (2010). Retrieved February 12, 2010, from http://www.thework.com/about.asp

[xxix] Dyer, W. (2004). *The Power of Intention.* Carlsbad: Hay House, Inc., 44

[xxx] Hendricks, G. (2009). *The Big Leap, Conquer Your Hidden fear and Take Life to the Next Level.* New York: Harper One., 20

[xxxi] Tolle, E. (2004). *The Power of Now: A Guide to Spiritual Enlightenment.* Vancouver: Namaste Publishing

[xxxii] Amen, D. G. (1998). *Change Your Brain Change Your Life, The Breakthrough Program for Conquering Anxiety, Depression, Obsessiveness, Anger and Impulsiveness.* New York: Three Rivers Press., 82-96

[xxxiii] Ibid., 186

[xxxiv] Ibid., 150-170

[xxxv] Ibid., 37-43

[xxxvi] Ibid., 273

[xxxvii] "The Honey Do List Strategy" used with permission from Love and Infertility: Survival Strategies for Balancing Infertility, Marriage and Life by Kristen Magnacca, pp 101-108

[xxxviii] "Keep Time In Perspective Strategy" Used with permission from Love and Infertility: Survival Strategies for Balancing Infertility, Marriage and Life by Kristen Magnacca, pp 123-127

[xxxix] Oprah Soul Series. (2009, June 10). Oprah interview will Jill Bolton Taylor. Retrieved February 12, 2010, from http://www.oprah.com/oprahradio/Jill-Bolte-Taylor-on-Oprahs-Soul-Series-Webcast

[xl] Marx Hubbard, B. (1998). *Conscious Evolution Awakening the Power of Our Social Potential.* Novato California: New World Library., 10

[xli] Dale, C. (2009). *The Subtle Body An Encyclopedia of Your Energetic Anatomy.* Boulder : Sounds True.,117

[xlii] Ibid., 28

[xliii] Institute of HeartMath. (2010). *Science of Coherence.* Retrieved February 12, 2010, from http://www.heartmath.org/research/overview.html

[xliv] Dale, C. (2009). *The Subtle Body An Encyclopedia of Your Energetic Anatomy.* Boulder : Sounds True., 27

[xlv] Ibid., 27

[xlvi] Ibid., 123

[xlvii] http://www.energeticnutrition.com/vitalzym/xeno_phyto_estrogens.html

---

[xlviii] Makichen, W. (2005). *Spirit Babies, How to Communicate with the Child You're Meant to Have.* New York: Delta Trade Paperbacks, 186-187
[xlix] Brown, M. (2005). *The Presence Process A Healing Journey Into Present Moment Awareness.* Vancouver: Namaste Publishing., 10
[l] Nhat Hanh, T. (2009). *Happiness: Essential Mindfulness* . Berkeley: Parallel Press, 3
[li] Ibid., 5
[lii] Ibid., 6
[liii] Schell, F., Allolio, B., & Schonecke, O. (2005). Physiological and psychological effects of Hatha yoga exercise in healthy women. *Journal of Psychosomatic Research, 41*, 46-52
[liv] Mate , G. (2003). *When the Body Says No: Understanding the Stress-Disease Connection.* Vancouver: John Wiley & Sons, Inc., 89-90
[lv] Domar, A., Clapp, D., Slawsby, E., Dusek, J., Kessel, B., & Freizinger, B. (2000). Impact of group psychological interventions on pregnancy rates in infertile women. Fertility and Sterility . *Fertility and Sterility* , *73*(4), 805-811
[lvi] *Fighting Infertility At The Chiropractor* (2004, February 25). Retrieved February 12, 2010, from http://www.chiro.org/research/FULL/Fighting_Infertility_At_The_Chiropractor.htm
[lvii] Fertility Massage (n.d.). Retrieved February 12, 2010, from http://gawain.membrane.com/fertility/fertility_massage.html

---

[lviii] Reflexology For Infertility (2007, March 17). Retrieved February 12, 2010, from http://infertility.suite101.com/article.cfm/reflexology_for_infertility
[lix] Andrea Perry. (n.d.). Is reflexology the new cure for infertility?. Retrieved February 12, 2010, from http://www.dailymail.co.uk/health/article-20980/Is-reflexology-new-cure-infertility.html
[lx] Doidge, N. (2007). *The Brain that Changes Itself, Stories of Personal Triumph from the Frontiers of Brain Science*. England: Penguin Books, 74
[lxi] Diego, M., Field, T., Sanders, C., & Hernandez-Reif, M. (2004). Massage therapy of moderate and light pressure and vibrator effects on EEG and heart rate. . *International Journal of Neuroscience, 114*, 31-44
[lxii] Arvigo, Rosita, Nadine Epstein, *Rainforest Home Remedies: The Maya Way to Heal Your Body and Replenish Your Soul* (New York: Harper Collins Publishers, 2001), 6
[lxiii] Ibid.,3
[lxiv] Ibid.,8
[lxv] Ibid.,32
[lxvi] Personal MD, Your lifeline online. (2000, March 23). Gynecologists Investigate Massage As Infertility Treatment. Retrieved February 12, 2010, from http://www.personalmd.com/news/n0323123924.shtml

---

[lxvii] Gregory, Catherine S. "Mayan Womb Massage: How an ancient technique can help prepare your body for conception and ease menstrual cramps," *Mothering,* March-April, 2010, 58

[lxviii] Arvigo, Rosita, Nadine Epstein, *Rainforest Home Remedies: The Maya Way to Heal Your Body and Replenish Your Soul* (New York: Harper Collins Publishers, 2001), 32

[lxix] Ibid.,14

[lxx] Ibid.,18

[lxxi] Ibid.,16

[lxxii] Ibid.,34

[lxxiii] Lewis, R. (2008). *Understanding Eastern Medicine and Fertility*. Retrieved February 12, 2010, from http://www.thefertilesoul.com/Methodology/Eastern%20Medicine/easternmedicine.aspx

[lxxiv] Dechar, L. E. (2004). Five Spirits: Tao. Retrieved February 12, 2010, from http://www.fivespirits.com/about.php

[lxxv] Unexplained Infertility: The Culprit Could Be Celiac Disease - Now Much Easier To Diagnose With A New Home Screening Test (2009, February 16). Retrieved February 12, 2010, from http://www.medicalnewstoday.com/articles/139159.php

[lxxvi] Joswick, Diana. "February Acupuncture Newsletter - Reproductive Health" www.acufinder.com. 10 Feb. 2009. <http://www.acufinder.com>.

---

[lxxvii] Manheimer, Eric, Grant Zhang, Laurence Udoff, Aviad Haramati, Patricia Langenberg, Brian M. Berman, and Lex M. Bouter. "Effects of acupuncture on rates of pregnancy and live birth among women undergoing in vitro fertilization: systematic review and meta-analysis." British Medical Journal (2008). BMJ medical publications of the year. 7 Feb. 2008. 9 Apr. 2009 <http://www.bmj.com/cgi/content/full/bmj.39471.430451.BEv1>

[lxxviii] Dieterle, Stefan, Gao Ying, Wolfgang Hatzmann, and Andreas Neuer. "Effect of acupuncture on the outcome of in vitro fertilization and intracytoplasmic sperm injection: a randomized, prospective, controlled clinical study." 7 Apr. 2006. 9 Apr. 2009 <http://www.ncbi.nlm.nih.gov/pubmed/16616748/>

[lxxix] Westergaard, Lars G. M.D., Ph.D, Mao, Qunhui M.D, Krogslund, Marianne, Sadrini, Steen, Lenz, Suzan M.D., Ph.D, Grinsted, Jorgen M.D., Ph.D. Acupuncture Improves pregnancy rates in IVF treatments. 2006

[lxxx] Udoff, L.C., G. Zhang, S. Patwardhan, Z. Wei, and H.D. McClamrock. "The effect of acupuncture on outcomes in in-vitro fertilization (IVF)." 20 Apr. 2006. 9 Apr. 2009 <http://clinicaltrials.gov/ct2/show/NCT00317317>

---

[lxxxi] Galch, Michael Reed. *Acupressure Potent Points A Guide to Self-Care for Common Ailments.* Bantam Books 1990

[lxxxii] Lewis, R. (2006). *Fertility Enhancing DVD Lecture Series, Session A: Nourishing Your Fertile Soul: Enhancing the Reproductive Response* . Asheville: The Fertile Soul

[lxxxiii] *What Health* (n.d.). Retrieved February 12, 2010, from http://whathealth.com/bmi/formula.html

[lxxxiv] Crosignani, P., Colombo, M., Vegetti, W., Somigliana, E., Gessati , A., & Ragni, G. (2003). Verweight and obese anovulatory patients with polycystic ovaries: parallel improvements in anthropometric indices, ovarian physiology and fertility rate induced by diet. *Human Reproduction, 18*(9), 1928-1932

[lxxxv] Simmons Flynn, K. (2009, May 31). Blood Sugar Balance: Manage Your Mood and Weight. Retrieved February 12, 2010, from http://www.fertilefoods.com/healthy-pregnancy/pregnancy/blood-sugar-balance-manage-your-mood-and-weight/

[lxxxvi] Simmons Flynn, K. (2010). *Cooking for Fertility: Foods to Nourish Your Fertile Soul.* Asheville: The Fertile Soul

[lxxxvii] Dellorto, Danielle. "Study: Caffeine may boost miscarriage risk." CNN.com/health. 21 Jan. 2008

[lxxxviii] Simmons Flynn, K. (2010). *Cooking for Fertility: Foods to Nourish Your Fertile Soul.* Asheville: The Fertile Soul.
[lxxxix] Ibid
[xc] Simmons Flynn, K. (2009, Feb 28). Wheat and Gluten Free Grains. Retrieved February 12, 2010, from http://www.fertilefoods.com/healthy-pregnancy/pregnancy/wheat-free-and-gluten-free-grains/
[xci] Ball, D., & Pollard, T. (2009, December 22). Ask the Doctor: Celiac disease verses non-celiac gluten sensitivity. Retrieved February 12, 2010, from http://community.eatingforevolution.com/articles/308
[xcii] Simmons Flynn, K. (2009, Apr 4). Cow Dairy Alternatives. Retrieved February 12, 2010, from http://www.fertilefoods.com/healthy-pregnancy/fertility/cow-dairy-alternatives/
[xciii] Willett, Walter C., Patrick J. Skerrett, and Jorge E. Chavarro. The Fertility Diet. New York: McGraw-Hill Companies, The, 2007; 73
[xciv] Simmons Flynn, K. (2009, Feb 15). Fertility Friendly Fast Food Alternatives. Retrieved February 12, 2010, from http://www.fertilefoods.com/healthy-pregnancy/fertility/fertility-friendly-fast-food-alternatives/

---

[xcv] Simmons Flynn, K. (2009, Feb 15). Mindful Eating. Retrieved February 12, 2010, from http://www.fertilefoods.com/healthy-pregnancy/pregnancy/mindful-eating/

[xcvi] Than, K. (2006, February 8). How Sperm Get Hyperactive . Retrieved February 12, 2010, from http://www.livescience.com/health/060208_hyper_sperm.html

[xcvii] Lipton, Ph.D. , B. H. (2002). Nature, Nurture and Human Development. Journal of Prenatal and Perinatal Psychology and Health, 16, 167-180. Retrieved February 12, 2010, from http://www.hofmann.org/papers/Lipton_Human%20Devel.html

[xcviii] Krohmer, Ph.D., R. W. (n.d.). The Reproductive System. Retrieved February 12, 2010, from http://www.scribd.com/doc/5012437/The-reproductive-system

[xcix] Northrup, M.D., C. (2006). *Women's Bodies, Women's Wisdom Creating Physical and Emotional Health and Healing*. New York: Bantam Books, 217

[c] Lewis, R. (2006). Egg Quality. Powerpoint Presentation, The Fertile Soul, Asheville

[ci] Northrup, M.D., C. (2006). Women's Bodies, Women's Wisdom Creating Physical and Emotional Health and Healing. New York: Bantam Books

---

[cii] Knowmycycle.com. (2008, August). Hormones and their Roles. Retrieved February 12, 2010, from http://www.knowmycycle.com/menstrual-hormones.aspx

[ciii] Simmons Flynn, K. (2009, Mar 7). Learning to Chart Your Menstrual Cycle for Conception. Retrieved February 12, 2010, from http://www.fertilefoods.com/healthy-pregnancy/fertility/learning-to-chart-your-menstrual-cycle/

[civ] Weschler, T. (2006). Taking Charge of Your Fertility. New York: Harper Collins

[cv] Bolton Taylor, J. (2006). My Stroke of Insight. New York: Penguin Group, 110

[cvi] Stewart, & et all (1991). Eating disorders from a gynecologic and endocrinologic view: hormonal changes. Fertility and Sterility, 81(4), 1151-1153

[cvii] In Vitro Fertilization IVF Find all about vitro . (n.d.). Medication that cause infertility. Retrieved February 12, 2010, from http://in-vitro-fertilization.eu/medication-and-toxic-substances-which-can-produce-infertility/

[cviii] Georgia Reproductive Specialists. (2007). Testing for Male Factor Infertility. Retrieved February 12, 2010, from http://www.ivf.com/maletesting.html

[cix] Center for Reproductive Medicine and Vasectomy Reversal. (2009). Retrieved February 12, 2010, from http://www.malereproduction.com/sperm_chromatin_structure.html

[cx] He, S., & Woods, III, L. (2004). Changes in motility, ultrastructure, and fertilization capacity of striped bass Morone saxatilis spermatozoa following cryopreservation. Retrieved February 12, 2010, from http://www.sciencedirect.com/science?_ob=ArticleURL&_udi=B6T4D-4C709MM-2&_user=10&_coverDate=06%2F14%2F2004&_rdoc=1&_fmt=high&_orig=search&_sort=d&_docanchor=&view=c&_searchStrId=1205174926&_rerunOrig

[cxi] Tartagni, M., Schonauer, M., Cicinelli, E., Selman, H., De Ziegler, D., Petruzzelli, F., et al. (2002). Usefulness of the Hypo-Osmotic Swelling Test in Predicting Pregnancy Rate and Outcome in Couples Undergoing Intrauterine Insemination. *Journal of Andrology*, 23(4). Retrieved February 12, 2010, from http://www.andrologyjournal.org/cgi/content/abstract/23/4/498

[cxii] Yamamoto , M. G., Hibi, H., Katsuno, S., & Miyaki, K. (1995). Serum estradiol levels in normal men and men with idiopathic infertility. *International Journal of Urology*, 2(1), 44-46.

---

[cxiii] Adelson, J., & Adelson, H. (1987). Serum estradiol levels in normal men and men with idiopathic infertility. *International Journal of Urology*, 2(1), 139-141
[cxiv] Bakalar, N. (2006, November 14). *Fertility: Iron Supplements May Reduce Risk of Infertility.* Retrieved February 12, 2010, from http://www.nytimes.com/2006/11/14/health/14fert.html?_r=1
[cxv] Dale, C. (2009). *The Subtle Body An Encyclopedia of Your Energetic Anatomy*. Boulder : Sounds True, 44
[cxvi] Better Health Channel. (2010, February 13). Congenital adrenal hyperplasia. Retrieved February 12, 2010, from http://www.betterhealth.vic.gov.au/bhcv2/bhcarticles.nsf/pages/Congenital_adrenal_hyperplasia
[cxvii] Better Health Channel. (2010, February 13). Cushing's Syndrome. Retrieved February 12, 2010, from http://www.betterhealth.vic.gov.au/bhcv2/bhcarticles.nsf/pages/Congenital_adrenal_hyperplasia
[cxviii] Epigee. (2009). *Chances of Pregnancy by Day of Intercourse day zero is ovulation*. Retrieved February 12, 2010, from http://www.epigee.org/health/infertility.html

---

[cxix] Raine-Fenning, N., Jayaprakasan, K., Chamberlain, S., Devlin , L., Priddle, H., & Johnson, I. (2009). Automated measurements of follicle diameter: a chance to standardize? . *Fertility and Sterility, 91*(4), 1469-1472
[cxx] Massey, D. (2009, November 12). *IVF and Antral Follicle Count*. Retrieved February 12, 2010, from http://cnyfertility.com/index.php?s=Verkagen
[cxxi] Weiss, R. (2003, May 8). 400,000 Human Embryos Frozen in U.S. Number at Fertility Clinics Is Far Greater Than Previous Estimates, Survey Finds. Retrieved February 12, 2010, from http://www.washingtonpost.com/ac2/wp-dyn?pagename=article&contentId=A27495-2003May7
[cxxii] Finch, C. E., & Rose, M. R. (1995). Ormones and the Physiological Architecture of Life History Evolution. The Quarterly Review of Biology, 70(1), 1-52. Retrieved February 12, 2010, from http://www.washingtonpost.com/ac2/wp-dyn?pagename=article&contentId=A27495-2003May7
[cxxiii] Lewis, R. (n.d.). *Advanced Maternal Age and Egg Quality* . Retrieved February 12, 2010, from hhttp://www.acudenver.com/articles/Articles RL1.pdf
[cxxiv] Ibid.

---

[cxxv] Northrup, M.D., C. (2006). *Women's Bodies, Women's Wisdom Creating Physical and Emotional Health and Healing*. New York: Bantam Books, 436-437
[cxxvi] Raymond, J. (2008, September 15). *Modern Maternity*. Retrieved February 12, 2010, from http://www.newsweek.com/id/158410
[cxxvii] OBGYN.net Publications. (n.d.). Endometriosis: A New Picture of the Disease is Emerging. Retrieved February 12, 2010, from http://www.obgyn.net/women/women.asp?page=/endo/marylou/ml004
[cxxviii] Laparoscopic Surgery for Infertile Women with Mild Endometriosis. (1997). *Journal Watch General Medicine*. Retrieved February 12, 2010, from http://general-medicine.jwatch.org/cgi/content/full/1997/725/1
[cxxix] (Morris, C. (n.d.). Endometriosis and Acupuncture. Retrieved February 12, 2010, from http://www.endo-resolved.com/acupuncture.html
[cxxx] Lewis, R. (2006). Understanding Your Diagnosis- Endometriosis. Retrieved February 12, 2010, from http://www.thefertilesoul.com/knowledgebase/diagnoses/diagnosisdetail.aspx?id=220.

---

[cxxxi] OBGYN.net Publications. (n.d.). Endometriosis: A New Picture of the Disease is Emerging. Retrieved February 12, 2010, from http://www.obgyn.net/women/women.asp?page=/endo/marylou/ml004

[cxxxii] Energetic Nutrition. (n.d.). Environmental Estrogens Xenoestrogens and Phytoestrogens. Retrieved February 12, 2010, from http://www.energeticnutrition.com/vitalzym/xeno_phyto_estrogens.html

[cxxxiii] Mate , G. (2003). *When the Body Says No: Understanding the Stress-Disease Connection*. Vancouver: John Wiley & Sons, Inc.

[cxxxiv] Northrup, M.D., C. (2006). *Women's Bodies, Women's Wisdom Creating Physical and Emotional Health and Healing*. New York: Bantam Books.,169-170

[cxxxv] Lewis, R. (2006). Understanding Your Diagnosis- Uterine Fibrosis. Retrieved February 12, 2010, from http://www.thefertilesoul.com/knowledgebase/diagnoses/diagnosisdetail.aspx?id=222

[cxxxvi] *Fibroid Massage Techniques* (n.d.). Retrieved February 12, 2010, from http://hubpages.com/hub/Fibroid-Massage-Techniques).

[cxxxvii] Myss, C. (1996). *Anatomy of the Spirit the Seven Stages of Power and Healing*, 109

---

[cxxxviii] "The Dream List" used with permission from Love and Infertility: Survival Strategies for Balancing Infertility, Marriage and Life by Kristen Magnacca, pp 4-9

[cxxxix] Royal College of Obstetricians and Gynaecologist. (2004, January). *Couples with recurrent miscarriage: What the RCOG guideline means for you*. Retrieved February 12, 2010, from http://www.rcog.org.uk/womens-health/clinical-guidance/couples-recurrent-miscarriage-what-rcog-guideline-means-you

[cxl] Ibid.

[cxli] Peterson, MD, C. (n.d.). *Recurrent miscarriage: What are the causes?*. Retrieved February 12, 2010

[cxlii] (Hereditary Thrombophilia and Thrombocythemia in Pregnancy (n.d.). Retrieved February 12, 2010, from http://www.femalepatient.com/html/arc/sig/case/articles/031_07_035.asp

[cxliii] Jauniaux, E., Farquharson, R., Christiansen, O., & Exalto, N. (2006). Evidence-based guidelines for the investigation and medical treatment of recurrent miscarriage . Human Reproduction, 1-7. Retrieved February 12, 2010, from http://humrep.oxfordjournals.org/cgi/reprint/del150v1.pdf

[cxliv] Jauniaux, E., Farquharson, R., Christiansen, O., & Exalto, N. (2006). Evidence-based guidelines for the investigation and medical treatment of recurrent miscarriage . Human Reproduction, 1-7. Retrieved February 12, 2010, from http://humrep.oxfordjournals.org/cgi/reprint/del150v1.pdf

[cxlv] Dellorto, Danielle. "Study: Caffeine may boost miscarriage risk." CNN.com/health. 21 Jan. 2008.
28 Oct. 2008.
http://www.cnn.com/2008/health/conditions/01/21hfh.caffeine.miscarriage/index.html

[cxlvi] The Arvigo Techniques of Maya Abdominal Massage Female Pelvic Anatomy and Physiology. Rosita Arvigo, 69

[cxlvii] Women's Bodies, Women's Wisdom Creating Physical and Emotional Health and Healing Christiane Northrup Bantam Books New York 2006, 453

[cxlviii] Makichen, W. (2005). *Spirit Babies, How to Communicate with the Child You're Meant to Have.* New York: Delta Trade Paperbacks, 92

[cxlix] DeBartolo Clinic. (2002). *DeBartolo PMS™ Nutritional Support For Menstrual Discomforts.* Retrieved February 12, 2010, from http://debartoloclinic.com/pms.htm

[cl] Lewis, R. (n.d.). *Clinical Study Detail*. Retrieved February 12, 2010, from http://www.thefertilesoul.com/knowledgebase/clinical/clinicalstudies.aspx?id=1832
[cli] Arvigo, R. (n.d.). *The Arvigo Techniques of Maya Abdominal Massage: Female Pelvic Anatomy and Physiology*, 99
[clii] Magnacca, K. (2004). *Love and Infertility Survival Strategies for Balancing Infertility, Marriage and Life*. Washington DC: Lifeline Press, 99
[cliii] Santa Cruz Natural Health. (2009, September). *New Studies Confirm Acupuncture Helps PCOS!*. Retrieved February 12, 2010, from http://www.santacruznaturalhealth.com/2009/09/new-studies-confirm-acupuncture-helps-pcos/
[cliv] Women's Health. (n.d.). *Acupuncture for PCOS*. Retrieved February 12, 2010, from (http://www.womens-health.co.uk/acupuncture.html
[clv] Ibid.
[clvi] Crosignani, P., Colombo, M., Vegetti, W., Somigliana, E., Gessati , A., & Ragni, G. (2003). Verweight and obese anovulatory patients with polycystic ovaries: parallel improvements in anthropometric indices, ovarian physiology and fertility rate induced by diet. *Human Reproduction*, *18*(9), 1928-1932

[clvii] *Usana Health Sciences- Nutritionals You Can Trust* (n.d.). Retrieved February 12, 2010, from http://www.cnyfertility.usana.com/

[clviii] Northrup, M.D., C. (2006). *Women's Bodies, Women's Wisdom Creating Physical and Emotional Health and Healing*. New York: Bantam Books, 101

[clix] International Premature Ovarian Failure Assoc. (n.d.). *Premature Ovarian Failure (POF) Fact Sheet*. Retrieved February 12, 2010, from http://www.pofsupport.org/information/factsheet/fact_sheet_english.pdf

[clx] Ibid.

[clxi] The Fertile Soul. (n.d.). *Scientific Evidence: Clinical Studies*. Retrieved February 12, 2010, from http://www.thefertilesoul.com/Knowledgebase/Clinical/clinical.aspx

[clxii] Diego, M. A., Field, T., Sanders, C., & Hernandez-Reif, M. (2004). Massage therapy of moderate and light pressure and vibrator effects on EEG and heart rate. International Journal of Neuroscience, 114, 31-44

[clxiii] Lewis, R. (n.d.). Mechanical Barriers to Conception: Tubal OBstructions, Pelvic Adhesions and Pelvic Inflammatory Disease (PID). Retrieved February 12, 2010, from http://www.thefertilesoul.com/knowledgebase/diagnoses/diagnosisdetail.aspx?id=228

[clxiv] Ibid.

---

[clxv] Personal MD. (2000, March 23). Gynecologists Investigate Massage As Infertility Treatment . Retrieved February 12, 2010, from http://www.personalmd.com/news/n0323123924.shtml

[clxvi] Fertility Massage (n.d.). Retrieved February 12, 2010, from http://gawain.membrane.com/fertility/fertility_massage.html

[clxvii] Wing, T., & Sedlmeier, E. (n.d.). Measuing the Effectiveness of Chinese Herbal Medicine in Improving Female Fertility. Retrieved February 12, 2010, from http://www.thefertilesoul.com/knowledgebase/clinical/clinicalstudies.aspx?id=962

[clxviii] Diego, M., Field, T., Sanders, C., & Hernandez-Reif, M. (2004). Massage therapy of moderate and light pressure and vibrator effects on EEG and heart rate. *International Journal of Neuroscience, 114*, 31-44